Reiki And Chakras

Self Help Guide for Healing Through Reiki, Achieve Spiritual Mindfulness, Awakening Chakras and Third Eye

(Awake Your Hidden Energy With Crystals)

David Lubeck

Published by Rob Miles

David Lubeck

All Rights Reserved

Reiki and Chakras: Self Help Guide for Healing Through Reiki, Achieve Spiritual Mindfulness, Awakening Chakras and Third Eye (Awake Your Hidden Energy With Crystals)

ISBN 978-1-989990-29-2

All rights reserved. No part of this guide may be reproduced in any form without permission in writing from the publisher except in the case of brief quotations embodied in critical articles or reviews.

Legal & Disclaimer

The information contained in this book is not designed to replace or take the place of any form of medicine or professional medical advice. The information in this book has been provided for educational and entertainment purposes only.

The information contained in this book has been compiled from sources deemed reliable, and it is accurate to the best of the Author's knowledge; however, the Author cannot guarantee its accuracy and validity and cannot be held liable for any errors or omissions. Changes are periodically made to this book. You must consult your doctor or get professional medical advice before using any of the suggested remedies, techniques, or information in this book.

Upon using the information contained in this book, you agree to hold harmless the Author from and against any damages, costs, and expenses, including any legal fees potentially resulting from the application of any of the information provided by this guide. This disclaimer applies to any damages or injury caused by the use and application, whether directly or indirectly, of any advice or information presented, whether for breach of contract, tort, negligence, personal injury, criminal intent, or under any other cause of action.

You agree to accept all risks of using the information presented inside this book. You need to consult a professional medical practitioner in order to ensure you are both able and healthy enough to participate in this program.

Table of Contents

INTRODUCTION 1

CHAPTER 1: STARTING YOUR JOURNEY 3

CHAPTER 2: HOW TO INCREASE YOUR POWER 21

CHAPTER 3: WHAT REIKI CAN DO FOR YOU 31

CHAPTER 4: WHAT IS REIKI? 42

CHAPTER 5: HOW TO START 47

CHAPTER 6: HISTORY OF REIKI 65

CHAPTER 7: REIKI ATTUNEMENT 78

CHAPTER 8: WHAT IS REIKI? 85

CHAPTER 9: HISTORY OF REIKI 90

CHAPTER 10: HOW REIKI BEGAN: THE HISTORY 109

CHAPTER 11: HISTORY OF REIKI 116

CHAPTER 12: PRINCIPLES OF REIKI PRACTICE 129

CHAPTER 13: REIKI CLOTHING 134

CHAPTER 14: REIKI PRINCIPLES: GETTING STARTED WITH THE FIVE PRINCIPLES 138

CHAPTER 15: BASIC REIKI HEALING TECHNIQUES 149

CHAPTER 16: CHAKRAS IN THE CONTEXT OF REIKI......... 158

CHAPTER 17: BREATHING: IT REALLY IS IMPORTANT!.... 170

CHAPTER 18: THE CHAKRAS, MERIDIANS AND ALSO REIKI 174

CHAPTER 19: OTHER SELF-HEALING TECHNIQUES.......... 193

CONCLUSION... 202

Introduction

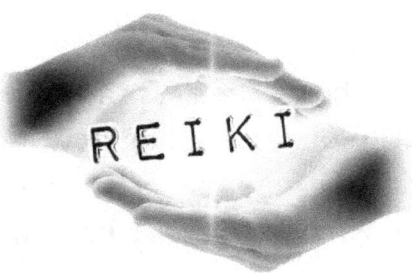

Have you ever wanted to learn about the practice of Reiki and discover the benefits and healing it can provide?

The power of Reiki and its powerful ability to soothe and heal the mind, soul, and body can transform the way you live and enjoy your life.

Learning about Reiki begins with an understanding of the practice and its purpose.

If you have considered Reiki as a form of treatment, you may know some of the principles involved with this practice.

Before you consider learning Reiki, you may want to experience the effects of its power through an online, distance treatment, or from a local master or practitioner.

Learning about Reiki is a journey that begins with understanding how it connects us with the energy or power of the universe, which is already present in all of us.

The key to understanding and developing Reiki is to harness and work with this energy for self-treatment and the healing of others.

Chapter 1: Starting Your Journey

Mindset

When beginning upon a new journey of any kind, it is important that you open yourself up for whatever path this may lead you down. Your journey toward spiritual enlightenment and becoming one with the life pulsing through the entirety of the universe is no different. In fact, this is an adventure of the most epic proportions. One that will require the most finely attuned mindset. One that may change your life forever. One that has the possibility to change the entire world based on your mind set.

When beginning on your path with reiki you may have discovered this art thinking it will be a solution to absolutely every problem you encounter. As a matter of fact, this may or may not be true. It is important to have appropriate expectations from the beginning however. While reiki may be able to have a huge impact on every element of your life and the world, your ability to manifest its creations will take a lot of time, effort, and practice. So for that reason, you should not go into reiki thinking you will be able to instantly fix all of the problems you see in your life.

While you are well on your way toward acquiring the knowledge and experience in order to use the art of reiki toward affecting all elements of your life, it is important to remember that this art is not the only tool with which to change your life and the world. This is not the only solution. This is merely one of many solutions. Part of understanding this healing is understanding that it is merely a piece in a larger puzzle. To truly affect your own life you must make changes across the board. Pulling the energy from the Earth will only manifests so much. But your ability to use mindfulness throughout the day, your chakras being aligned at all times, and the aura you presents to the world are all elements of change as well. Much like starting a diet without adding exercise to your daily routine, you will only see very minimal results. However, once you integrate both diet and exercise into your life, you will see exponentially greater results. Using reiki along with other techniques such as crystals, chakra balancing, and mindfulness, you will see what a vast collection of tools can do to make a huge difference in the world.

Knowing that, you must begin your education with a beginner's mind. A beginner's mind is the idea that you are humbling yourself before knowledge that you do not yet possess. This beginner's mind is going to be crucial throughout your entire journey. This will neither be your first nor your last act of humbling yourself before a greater force. reiki itself is humbling because you are using the force of the entire universe, so admitting that you do not understand it is an ongoing fact from here on out. To truly appreciate the art, you will be learning you must not only admit that you do not know what you do not know, but you also must be appreciative of the fact that you do not know this, that you are learning this, and that there will always be more to learn. Rather than feeling shame, guilt, or fear around your ignorance or lack of knowledge, you must actually put yourself in the position to recognize that this is not a flaw but, in fact, it is the reason for your future success.

Energy

For the art of healing via reiki to truly occur there needs to be consensual giving and acceptance of this energy. To use the laying on of hands to conduct energy and move energy is not something that can be done successfully without your permission. Even when working on yourself, you have to create an area of consciousness in order to begin performing, but you also must create an area of consciousness around your own receiving of this energy. You must truly believe that you have the power to channel the universe's energy, and you must also believe that you are worthy of healing yourself.

It is not uncommon to have a mental block around the feelings of worthiness and acceptance for oneself. The idea of being able to heal another person is admirable because you're you are in service to another. However, the idea of healing oneself might bring up very deep emotional reservations for a lot of people. What a mighty power it is to be able to heal oneself. What a mighty thing to be in one with the universe. What a magnificent gift it is to give to yourself to use the life force of the world around you in order to heal yourself. You must want to be one with the universe in order to use its life force to heal yourself. This is a grand responsibility, but one you are already a part of, so it is truly best to take your own role in it seriously.

This acceptance is necessary because you are trying to cure areas that are restricted. As discussed earlier, energy is flowing in through and around all living and non-living objects on the Earth. That means it is flowing with or without your conscious awareness of it. Reiki is bringing your attention to it. So simply being unaware does not mean that everything is flowing freely and successfully on its own. No, in fact, once you bring your consciousness and awareness to the areas that are causing you pain, you will realize there are things restricting the energy from flowing through these places. The reason the pain is there is because there is an in balance. Once you take this education upon yourself you will have a responsibility to help alleviate some of these difficulties, whether in yourself or in two others.

Education

You have already begun your education in the art of healing with reiki. However, it is not a skill that you will master overnight. This is not a theoretical concept that can be fully comprehended by simply reading a book. While reading this book and learning from it is absolutely a necessary part of it, real learning will happen when you practice it. The art of laying hands is, unsurprisingly, a hands-on activity. You must absolutely try, practice, and possibly even fail before you succeed.

As discussed with the four different levels in the first chapter, to become the highest level of reiki master you must go through all four levels. However, if you are not interested in teaching others to use reiki, you do not have to complete all four levels of training. In fact, you can go through however many different levels you want, because there is no end goal in mind. Every person's journey will be different, and therefore every person's education will be unique to them.

Depending on how you go about completing the different levels of training, these could take anywhere from a few hours to years of training. While you may be able to go to a class or seminar in person that last simply one afternoon, this does not mean that you will be ready to move on to the next level the moment you are finished with that class. Most reiki practitioners encourage their students to take days, weeks, and months in between completing the various levels of education. This is because the power you are learning to work with is overwhelming, and it may take your body some time to adjust to the forces you are attempting to channel and manipulate. Much like beginning a new workout routine, you are muscles may be sore for a few days afterwards. As with reiki, when you are learning new techniques and abilities, it may take a while for your body to adjust and become settled with your new skills.

The farther along the levels you travel in your education of reiki will most likely increase exponentially the amount of time you spend in each level. Because level two is a more intense education than level one, it will most likely take you longer to complete level two, as well as taking you longer to settle into and recover from your education of the second degree before moving on to the third degree. If you do move all the way through all four levels to become a reiki master, this will almost certainly take you years. Do not be discouraged. Time will pass either way, so putting your time to good use and educating yourself in this magnificent practice is a glorious way to celebrate the time you have been given.

After you have completed reading this book, if you truly wants to be a conduit for reiki, you can find a reiki master in person. The reason for this is that even with all of the knowledge that this book possesses, the practice you will have acquired by attempting the upcoming instructions, and the altered mindset and understanding of what it takes to use reiki, the ability to use reiki must be given to you through a personal interaction with a reiki master-- either in person or via distance. This specific action is called attunement, and it is a necessary step in order to be given the ability to practice reiki. So an important step after you have finished reading this book is to either find a good reiki master near you, or simply ask the universe for a reiki master to attune you so that you will be able to really begin your practice.

Commitment

As with any new practice you want to incorporate into your life, the only way that it will become an integral and important part of your life is if you make a commitment to it. If you want to use the art of healing successfully and integrate it into your everyday life, you need to make space and time in every day to practice it. The most important things in your life should have priority. And what can be more important than bettering yourself in all sorts of ways. Whether you already have a practice of meditating, doing yoga, journaling, or working out, this is another aspect of taking care of yourself in order to be the best version of you today and in the future.

So the first part of committing is deciding how much you want to commit. Although every day is certainly a great ideal, if you do not think that this is a commitment you can actually put on your schedule and achieve, then this is not a promise you will want to make to yourself. You do not want to tell yourself you will do it every day and then beat yourself up if you do not get around to it. Decide how many days a week you want to begin focusing on your practice. You do not need large chunks of time. These do not have to be unmanageable events on your calendar.

Perhaps you want to spend 30 minutes three days a week. Find your daily schedule and block out a time for it. Perhaps you want to spend five minutes a day, every day. Make sure you know what time exactly those five minutes will occur, or you will not be committing to it.

There is no best schedule for anyone, nor is there any best time of day to work on it. The absolute best schedule for working on your reiki is at whatever frequency and whatever time is best for you to actually do it. Perhaps you want to begin your day with it, in which case maybe you want to practice reiki yourself first thing in the morning. Or maybe you have difficulty getting to sleep at night and therefore you could use this focus just before bed. Maybe you need a midday break during a stressful work day and there for a lunchtime routine would work best for you. There is no judgement or preferences outside of what works best for you. In fact, you might very well find that all three are what work best for you.

Prepare

Finally, before you get started with even your very first reiki session, you want to be physically and mentally prepared. Every single person will be different, so exactly what you may need varies from person to person, however, there are few things everyone can do to best get ready for the journey they are about to embark upon.

You are going to want to be the best mindset that you can put yourself in. This means that in order to stay focused and not get distracted you will want to have eaten a small meal about half an hour before you get started. You do not want to eat anything heavy, as this is more likely to make you sleepy. Nor do you want to eat anything that is especially difficult to digest, as you will very likely be distracted by that. Nor do you want to be especially thirsty throughout your session. You should have some water before hand, but not so much that you will need to use the restroom frequently throughout. It is advisable to avoid caffeine, as this is going to alter your natural state. Along those same lines you are not going to want to be under the influence of recreational drugs or alcohol. These will all alter the energy already flowing through you, thereby changing the very thing which you are trying to work on.

It is important to be rested for your session, because you do not want to become so sleepy that you fall asleep during the relaxing reiki session. It is also important that you use the time before your session to try to clear your mind of any outside distractions. Rather than thinking about what has already happened in your day or what is still left on your to-do list, this is a time to focus on the present and possibly even reflect on why you were at this juncture in the first place, and perhaps what you hope to get out of this journey.

It is very important for your reiki session that you are comfortable. If you are constantly fidgeting with a pair of pants that digs into your hips, or have your hair tied so tightly that it is giving you a headache, these are all going to be not only major distractions, but also they are going to alter the energy that you are trying to work with. Some things to consider are what you're wearing, as well as the temperature. Be ready to have layers to add or subtract in order to adjust accordingly to help cool or warm yourself, depending upon what your location is.

If you are working with a reiki master, you are going to want to ask them if they have any suggestions, recommendations, or rules about how you should prepare beforehand. A lot of practitioners have very specific rules such as: eliminating meat from your diet in the days leading up to your first session, going on a juice cleanse, eliminating alcohol for a few days prior, eliminating smoking from your days leading up to your session, possibly even going on a media diet of avoiding any outside media consumption, and in some cases, spending a good portion of time prior to your session in silence and solitude.

You should also ask what to expect before going into your first session. Most likely the space you will be in will be a quiet, calm, and inviting space. There may or may not be music, white noise, or silence. If you have a preference, it is absolutely appropriate to voice these to your reiki master, but there is also a good chance they have a reason for their own preference, so feel free to ask them about that. If you will be receiving reiki from them, you will probably do so while laying down, however, it can also certainly be done sitting or standing. This should happen while you are fully clothed and comfortable in your surroundings. This is going to include them putting their hands on and near your body. However, you should absolutely always feel safe enough to discuss with your reiki master exactly what you do and do not feel appropriate. Under no circumstances should it hurt or feel uncomfortable to you. If you have any areas of concern, perhaps you have an injury, perhaps you are especially ticklish, or perhaps you certain simply do not want to be touched in a certain spot, this is something you can and should share with them. If they are not receptive to any of this information, you should not practice with them.

To that end, there are also a few things you should do the following your first session, and therefore be prepared for before you even begin. Much like the preparations, these things include many of the same suggestions, but include more reflection. Some reiki Masters will ask you to do a three, seven, or even twenty one day cleanse of many of the aforementioned things such as alcohol, smoking, meat, and media. There will likely be a lot of thoughts and reflections happening, so being prepared with a journal is a good idea. And of course being well-rested, well hydrated, and well-nourished is an important part in your health, healing, and newly budding reiki practice

Chapter 2: How To Increase Your

Power

Be in a quiet, meditative place without interruptions.Let go of any thoughts, and allow yourself to just FEEL good – feel the blissful connection to Source, to God, to Goddess, that you likely remember having felt before, feel it now.Visualize the space around you filled with sparkling, euphoric, blissful, love-filled, light, the energy of The Creator, the energy of Source. Know that you are also made up of this same energy, just as everything in the entire universe is pure energy in its essence.

Be aware of the 3 feet of space in all directions around you, which is the boundary of your own energy space, the edge of the energy that is you - a large cocoon-shaped space of energy, 3 feet in all directions.

Own it powerfully, be it intensely, and fill that space up with as much awareness and strength and power and intensity and density of being YOU that you can imagine!!Focus for at least 60 seconds on making the energy space that is you, as densely filled with your being and your energy, as you can imagine – make the light be as thick as gel.

Then, be aware of the room that you are in, and expand into the room, and fill ALL of the room with the same level of awareness and strength and power and intensity and density of being YOU that you can imagine!! Feel what it's like to touch that cold hard corner of the ceiling, BE the whole room, fill it with YOU as thick as gel. NOW, bring ALL of that energy which just filled the room, back into just the 3-feet cocoon-like energy space that is YOU. Notice how much stronger you feel, that you're lighter, more confident, more connected to Source. Next, expand into TWO rooms, fill them BOTH with that same level of awareness and strength and power and intensity and density of being YOU that you can imagine.

Feel what it's like to touch that piece of furniture in the next room, or the lamp fixture on the ceiling of this room, BE the whole of both rooms, fill them with YOU as thick as gel. NOW, bring ALL of THAT energy back into just the 3-feet cocoon-like energy space that is YOU. Notice how you feel even more powerful, more strong, even more light, more confident, more connected to Source!!You can keep expanding to your whole apartment (or house), then back to your 3-foot space, then your whole block, and back to your 3-foot space, then your whole neighborhood, and back to your 3-foot space, etc.You can keep this up until you're filling the planet, the solar system, the galaxy, etc.

You will find this very effective and powerful.

How to Love and connect with your Inner Child

Sometimes we are aware if the feelings that weren't loved enough when we were very young in those years when our personality was being formed and solidified. This exercise allows you to go back in time and bring that missing love to your 5-year old self. This works because, in truth, time does not exist, we can change the past, change our perceptions. Be in a quiet, meditative place without interruptions.

Let go of any thoughts, and allow yourself to just FEEL good – feel the blissful connection to Source, to God, to Goddess, that you likely remember having felt before, feel it now. Sit in a chair, hold a pillow in your lap. Then, visualize, and FEEL, the pillow as 5-yr old YOU, on your lap, hold her in your arms, put your cheek gently down on the top of his head, say to her "I love you", say it with passion, FEEL how precious and innocent and sweet you were at that age, feel yourself as that beautiful little one, say to yourself "you are so beautiful, baby, you are precious, so pure, so sweet, so gentle, wanting so much just to be loved. Say to yourself, with so much passion, feeling, power and depth as you can allow yourself to feel.

Benefits and Limits of Reiki

Reiki is said to have multiple benefits and is applied for different needs, especially for clearing and tuning the chakras. One person may have a Reiki session to find relaxation from stress. A cancer patient might receive Reiki as a way to receive healing from the source. Some believe this energy comes from a higher power while others feel it comes from within. Despite these differences, many have experienced healing and the positive effects of Reiki.

Relieves pain, anxiety and fatigue

According to a review of randomized trials, reiki may help to reduce pain and anxiety, though more research is needed. It may also help to reduce fatigue. A 2015 study found that people being treated for cancer who received distant reiki in addition to regular medical care had lower levels of pain, anxiety, and fatigue. The use of reiki had been compared to physiotherapy for relieving lower back pain in people with herniated disk, both treatments were found to be equally effective at relieving back pains but reiki was more cost-effective and in some cases resulted in faster treatment.

Treats depression

Reiki treatments may be used as part of a treatment plan to help relieve depression. Researchers looked at the effects of reiki on older adults experiencing pain, depression, or anxiety and it reported an improvement on ones symptoms, mood and well-being. Reiki also brings about more feelings of relaxation, increased curiousity and enhances level of self-care.

Enhances quality of life

The positive benefits of reiki can enhance your overall well-being. Researchers has found out that reiki was helpful in improving the quality of life for women with cancer. Women who had reiki showed improvements to their sleep patterns, self-confidence, and depression levels. They noted a sense of calm, inner peace, and relaxation.

Boost moods

Reiki may help to improve your mood by relieving anxiety and depression. People who had reiki felt greater mood benefits compared to people who didn't have reiki. Reiki participants in a study who had six 30-minute sessions over a period of two to eight weeks showed improvements in their mood.

May improve some symptoms and conditions: Reiki may also be used to treat

❖ Headache

- ❖ Tension

- ❖ Insomnia

- ❖ Nausea

The relaxation response that happens with Reiki may benefit these symptoms. However, specific research is needed to determine the efficacy of reiki for the treatment of these symptoms and conditions.

May improve Memory and Behaviour

Reiki sessions has helped to improve the Behaviour and memory of people as a study that involves 24 patients with mild cognitive impairment and or and mild alzheimer's disease were carried out and reiki helped to improve their behavior greatly.

Reiki speeds up recovery from surgery or long-term illness

As it helps in adjusting to medicine/treatment, it also tends to reduce side-effects. For example, Chemotherapy patients who received Reiki noticed a marked decrease in side effects from treatment.

Reiki can be an effective way to treat immediate problems

such as physical or mental illness (recovery from surgery, but regular treatments can also improve overall health. By helping to maintain a state of physical and emotional balance, Reiki can not only treat problems, but perhaps even prevent them from ever developing.

Limitations of Reiki

Just like the benefits of reiki there are also limitations, the limitations sometimes isn't through the lack of power but by the lack of imagination on the parts of some practitioners. Imagination is both creative and experimental; a part of the mind that we use used to develop theories and ideas which are vital to our development in the way we accomplish what we already know whilst developing new ways of doing things. The limits of reiki are stated below;

❖ Recipients absence or lack of receptiveness

❖ Channel could be limited to begin with, although channels get stronger with time and practice

❖ Regular sessions are desirable

❖ Cannot give distance treatment

❖ Needs other treatment in addition to reiki incase of serious illness

❖ Deliberate refusal of healing

❖ Should not be applied as sole treatment in acute emergencies but it's an excellent support in emergency nterventions

❖ Will need other form of treatments in addition to reiki in cases of serious illness

❖ Incase regular sessions are not possible the effect may not be very prominent

Chapter 3: What Reiki Can Do For You

Until now we did not know the full story about Dr Usui due to not enough information coming from Japan, but this is changing. We now know that manuscripts from him and a couple of master's that he trained have been found and soon they will be shared with the western world. Also symbols that are used in Usui reiki are very similar to symbols found in a temple on Mount Karuna. These symbols came into his mind when he was on a 21-day retreat on Mount Karuna. Throughout his education, Dr. Usui had an interest in medicine, psychology and theology. As he was a learned man who had been a public servant, Industrialist, Politicians secretary, missionary and a Tendai monk amongst other things and travelled to western countries and China, it is likely that he picked up a lot of information on his travels and brought them all together and this all came together on the mountain and became Usui reiki – named after him. It is also believed that other styles of reiki were being practised in Japan around the same time.

Dr Usui opened a clinic in Japan to treat people either for free or at a low cost. His work became more publicised after an earthquake in 1923 where over 140,000 people were killed. He then worked very hard with his helpers to help as many people as they possibly could. One of his helpers was a man called Chujiro Hayashi. It is believed that he was the person who came up with the hand positions for giving a treatment. We know that it does not matter where your hands are laid, either on or above the body, as the energy will go to where it is needed. When being taught this way, it helps the students to be aware of where the Chakras are (energy points) so that they can learn to get more information from the body. The chakras are like spinning wheels and when the body is out of sorts, they can become sluggish and make you feel unwell. Reiki can help realign the chakras, helping people to become more balanced. I have many times had it shown to me that clients still feel as if my hands are on one place on the body when I have already moved on. They are even more amazed if they feel me at one end, and when they open their eyes, see me at the opposite side of them. The energy works with what the body needs.

Reiki can help to bring balance to the mind and emotions and helps give a feeling of wellbeing on all levels. Reiki is safe and natural and is now used in many hospitals all over the world. It can be used for pregnant women, the elderly, babies and animals. The energy can also be used on food, drinks and plants. In fact, it has unlimited uses and can be used in all situations. It can also give people a zest for living and help them make the changes to have a more positive outlook in life. I have had students getting watches and clocks to start working again after learning reiki. I always remember my teacher advising he was in a car with a student and the car broke down. After pulling up the bonnet and trying different things he got back in the car defeated. His student then suggested they used reiki on the car. The student teaching the teacher! We are all learning constantly. Guess what? After using reiki, he put the key in the ignition, and it started first time.

A reiki therapist cannot claim to heal any illness, but the energy will work with the body and mind to give what it needs at that point in time. One of my pet hates is if people call me a Healer. The energy is the healer and the person is only a conduit to allow the energy to access the body. It can also give those that are about to pass over a peaceful transition through acceptance. Reiki is now used in many hospitals and hospices across the world. It is good to see it becoming more mainstream. There have been scientific experiments done which show when someone is giving reiki, the client's energy levels increase to the same higher vibration as the therapist. More and more times in recent years I see published articles that show how reiki is being used in controlled settings and having great outcomes.

Seeing Reiki in action

Reiki can be given either seated or lying down. It can even be sent over distance. There is no reason to disrobe. I would suggest removing shoes and glasses and making yourself comfortable. Some people like to listen to music during a therapy session, others prefer silence. There is no one way that fits all. Sometimes people want to talk about what they are feeling either physically or emotionally. At other times people will be so relaxed that they will fall asleep. The important thing here is to go with what you, as a client, wish. I often find the birds outside my house joining in and so many people have said they like the bird music. The other interesting thing is if I hear a noise such as a fire engine going past, and at the end of the session I apologise for the noise, many times clients have been so chilled out they have not heard any external noises at all.

A year or so after being my friend's guinea pig I was co-ordinating a reiki workshop for a social group called SPICE. You should check this group out as it is UK wide. It stands for Special Programme of Initiative, Challenge and Excitement. During this evening, the Reiki Master had everyone sitting on chairs with our hands touching the shoulders of the people in front of us. There were about 6 rows of us. He then touched the first person gently. Within minutes people were saying they had heat, coldness, tingling or other sensations in areas where they had health problems. All I heard was "I had heat in my shoulder, I had a cold feeling in my knee, I had tingling in my foot". We were amazed that the energy was so strong that it was going through everyone by him touching only one person!

Later, that evening, after I had tidied away the chairs and everyone had left, I stopped to speak to him. I had a bad back problem and after sitting in the hard chair for three hours I was in agony. It was winter, and I had on warm clothes and my Jacket as I was ready to leave. He asked if I had a few minutes to sit down which I did. He then put his hands on my back, and I felt heat going through my Jacket. Through the heat, I felt my back-pain lessening until it disappeared completely. I was completely blown away. After suffering from back problems for over ten years, here was something that could help me. I was hooked!

My True Teacher

I decided after that evening to be trained in Reiki. I went for a couple of sessions with this teacher and then booked in a date to be trained to Level One Usui Reiki. An interesting thing happened on one of my visits for a therapy session though. I had taken a friend with me and she was sitting in the corner of the room. On this occasion I was feeling nothing and then I heard a sound coming from her corner. The energy had decided to work on her rather than me! She had Crystals in her pocket and felt the energy coming to her. It was so strong it was making her gasp. The reiki master advised that she must have needed it more than me. As you can guess I was a little upset as I had paid for the session. We soon had a laugh about it. I now know it is better to go in alone.

I could hardly contain my excitement as it got closer to the date of my workshop. I then received a phone call to advise me that not enough people had signed up for the workshop in my home town of

Edinburgh and would I like to go to one an hour away in Glasgow on a different date? I was devastated as I wanted neither of these. I had in my mind the date I was to be attuned and it had to be local to me. I had no idea at the time why I was feeling this way, but more was to become clearer as I went down this path.

Thinking of my friend I went and asked her who her teacher was and then called him. Unbelievably he was having a workshop on the date I had already pencilled in my diary to learn level one. Synchronicity at its best! He also only had another two people that he was training that day. I immediately thought this was a sign, as he did not cancel for small numbers and agreed to be trained by him. It was the best decision of my life and I owe the way my life has progressed to him. The day was fantastic. I remember giving a total stranger (one of the other students) reiki and felt the energy going to a part of his body. He advised this was an area where he had an ongoing problem. He was astonished, as was I, when he pinpointed an old injury I had as well. I was so excited after this day that I couldn't wait to try it out on others. I remember going home and it felt like I could not get the reiki to switch on. I felt sad thinking maybe I was only going to be able to do it at David's' house. Maybe there was something magical about it that I did not have in my home. I have since heard this from others so believe it must just be coming down from all the energy of the day. I did sleep well that night.

With any reiki training you have a twenty-one-day cleansing period to practise on yourself. A lot of changes can take place during this time which can include problems that you have buried in the past coming back to be resolved. I sometimes find that people can feel down for a few days then they experience an enormous high. They then tell me that they feel so positive and calm, so the few days were worth it. Others just sail through the process feeling fantastic from day one. I recently found my write up of my cleansing period. It was interesting looking back on how I was after my level one training. I had a few off days, then felt as if the world was a much brighter place to live in.

Chapter 4: What Is Reiki?

Reiki is a Japanese method for stress lessening and unwinding that also advances healing. It is administered by "lying on hands" and depends on the thought that a concealed "life power energy" courses through us and is what causes us to be alive. If one's "life power vitality" is low, then we will probably become ill or feel stress, and if it is high, we are more equipped for being cheerful and healthy.

The word Reiki is made of two Japanese words - Reid which signifies "God's Wisdom or the Higher Power" and Kid which is "life force energy". So Reiki is really "spiritually guided life force energy."

A treatment feels like a magnificent glowing brilliance that courses through and around you. Reiki treats the entire individual including body, feelings, mind and spirit creating numerous helpful impacts that include unwinding and feelings of peace, security and wellbeing. Numerous have reported extraordinary results.

Reiki is a basic, characteristic and safe method of spiritual healing and self-change that everyone can utilize. It has been powerful in helping for all intents and purposes every known disease and illness and dependably makes a valuable impact. It also works in conjunction with all other restorative or therapeutic methods to ease reactions and advance recovery.

An amazingly easy strategy to take in, the ability to utilize Reiki is not taught in the standard sense, but rather is exchanged to the understudy during a Reiki class. This ability is gone on during an "attunement" given by a Reiki ace and permits the understudy to take advantage of an unlimited supply of "life power energy" to enhance one's health and improve the quality of life.

Its utilization is not subject to one's intellectual capacity or spiritual advancement and therefore is accessible to everyone. It has been effectively taught to thousands of people of all ages and foundations.

While Reiki is spiritual in nature, it is not a religion. It has no creed, and there is nothing you should have faith so as to learn and utilize Reiki. Indeed, Reiki is not reliant on conviction at all and will work whether you have confidence in it or not. Since Reiki originates from God, numerous people find that using Reiki puts them more in contact with the experience of their religion rather than having just an intellectual idea of it.

While Reiki is not a religion, it is still essential to live and act in a way that advances agreement with others. Mikado Usual, the organizer of the Reiki arrangement of characteristic healing, prescribed that one practice certain basic moral standards to advance peace and amicability, which are nearly all inclusive over all societies.

During a meditation quite a while in the wake of developing Reiki, Mikado Usual chose to add the Reiki Ideals to the act of Reiki. The Ideals came to some degree from the five principles of the Meiji head of Japan whom Mikado Usual respected. The Ideals were produced to add spiritual equalization to Usual Reiki. Their motivation is to people understand that healing the spirit by intentionally deciding to enhance oneself is an essential part of the Reiki healing knowledge. All together for the Reiki healing energies to have lasting results, the customer must acknowledge responsibility for her or his healing and take a dynamic part in it. Therefore, the usual arrangement of Reiki is more than the utilization of the Reiki vitality. It should also include a dynamic commitment to enhance oneself all together for it to be a finished framework. The goals are both guidelines for living a thoughtful life and ethics deserving of practice for their inherent quality.

Chapter 5: How To Start

Mindset

When beginning upon a new journey of any kind, it is important that you open yourself up for whatever path this may lead you down. Your journey toward spiritual enlightenment and becoming one with the life pulsing through the entirety of the universe is no different. In fact, this is an adventure of the most epic proportions. One that will require the most finely attuned mindset. One that may change your life forever. One that has the possibility to change the entire world based on your mindset.

When beginning on your path with Reiki you may have discovered this art thinking it will be a solution to absolutely every problem you encounter. As a matter of fact, this may or may not be true. It is important to have appropriate expectations from the beginning, however. While Reiki may be able to have a huge impact on every element of your life and the world, your ability to manifest its creations will take a lot of time, effort, and practice. So for that reason, you should not go into Reiki thinking you will be able to instantly fix all of the problems you see in your life.

While you are well on your way toward acquiring the knowledge and experience in order to use the art of Reiki toward affecting all elements of your life, it is important to remember that this art is not the only tool with which to change your life and the world. This is not the only solution. This is merely one of many solutions. Part of understanding this healing is understanding that it is merely a piece in a larger puzzle. To truly affect your own life you must make changes across the board. Pulling the energy from the Earth will only manifests so much. But your ability to use mindfulness throughout the day, your chakras being aligned at all times, and the aura you present to the world are all elements of change as well. Much like starting a diet without adding exercise to your daily routine, you will only see very minimal results. However, once you integrate both diet and exercise into your life, you will see exponentially greater results. Using Reiki along with other techniques such as crystals, chakra balancing, and mindfulness, you will see what a vast collection of tools can do to make a huge difference in the world.

Knowing that, you must begin your education with a beginner's mind. A beginner's mind is the idea that you are humbling yourself before knowledge that you do not yet possess. This beginner's mind is going to be crucial throughout your entire journey. This will neither be your first nor your last act of humbling yourself before a greater force. Reiki itself is humbling because you are using the force of the entire universe, so admitting that you do not understand it is an ongoing fact from here on out. To truly appreciate the art, you will be learning you must not only admit that you do not know what you do not know, but you also must be appreciative of the fact that you do not know this, that you are learning this, and that there will always be more to learn. Rather than feeling shame, guilt, or fear around your ignorance or lack of knowledge, you must actually put yourself in the position to recognize that this is not a flaw but, in fact, it is the reason for your future success.

Energy

For the art of healing via Reiki to truly occur there needs to be consensual giving and acceptance of this energy. To use the laying on of hands to conduct energy and move energy is not something that can be done successfully without your permission. Even when working on yourself, you have to create an area of consciousness in order to begin performing, but you also must create an area of consciousness around your own receiving of this energy. You must truly believe that you have the power to channel the universe's energy, and you must also believe that you are worthy of healing yourself.

It is not uncommon to have a mental block around the feelings of worthiness and acceptance for oneself. The idea of being able to heal another person is admirable because you're you are in service to another. However, the idea of healing oneself might bring up very deep emotional reservations for a lot of people. What a mighty power it is to be able to heal oneself. What a mighty thing to be in one with the universe. What a magnificent gift it is to give to yourself to use the life force of the world around you in order to heal yourself. You must want to be one with the universe in order to use its life force to heal yourself. This is a grand responsibility, but one you are already a part of, so it is truly best to take your own role in it seriously.

This acceptance is necessary because you are trying to cure areas that are restricted. As discussed earlier, energy is flowing in through and around all living and non-living objects on the Earth. That means it is flowing with or without your conscious awareness of it. Reiki is bringing your attention to it. So simply being unaware does not mean that everything is flowing freely and successfully on its own. No, in fact, once you bring your consciousness and awareness to the areas that are causing you pain, you will realize there are things restricting the energy from flowing through these places. The reason the pain is there is because there is an in balance. Once you take this education upon yourself you will have a responsibility to help alleviate some of these difficulties, whether in yourself or in two others.

Education

You have already begun your education in the art of healing with Reiki. However, it is not a skill that you will master overnight. This is not a theoretical concept that can be fully comprehended by simply reading a book. While reading this book and learning from it is absolutely a necessary part of it, real learning will happen when you practice it. The art of laying hands is, unsurprisingly, a hands-on activity. You must absolutely try, practice, and possibly even fail before you succeed.

As discussed with the four different levels in the first chapter, to become the highest level of Reiki master you must go through all four levels. However, if you are not interested in teaching others to use Reiki, you do not have to complete all four levels of training. In fact, you can go through however many different levels you want, because there is no end goal in mind. Every person's journey will be different, and therefore every person's education will be unique to them.

Depending on how you go about completing the different levels of training, these could take anywhere from a few hours to years of training. While you may be able to go to a class or seminar in person that last simply one afternoon, this does not mean that you will be ready to move on to the next level the moment you are finished with that class. Most Reiki practitioners encourage their students to take days, weeks, and months in between completing the various levels of education. This is because the power you are learning to work with is overwhelming, and it may take your body some time to adjust to the forces you are attempting to channel and manipulate. Much like beginning a new workout routine, you are muscles may be sore for a few days afterward. As with Reiki, when you are learning new techniques and abilities, it may take a while for your body to adjust and become settled with your new skills.

The farther along the levels you travel in your education of Reiki will most likely increase exponentially the amount of time you spend in each level. Because level two is a more intense education than level one, it will most likely take you longer to complete level two, as well as taking you longer to settle into and recover from your education of the second degree before moving on to the third degree. If you do move all the way through all four levels to become a Reiki master, this will almost certainly take you years. Do not be discouraged. Time will pass either way, so putting your time to good use and educating yourself in this magnificent practice is a glorious way to celebrate the time you have been given.

After you have completed reading this book, if you truly want to be a conduit for Reiki, you can find a Reiki master in person. The reason for this is that even with all of the knowledge that this book possesses, the practice you will have acquired by attempting the upcoming instructions, and the altered mindset and understanding of what it takes to use Reiki, the ability to use Reiki must be given to you through a personal interaction with a Reiki master--either in person or via distance. This specific action is called attunement, and it is a necessary step in order to be given the ability to practice Reiki. So an important step after you have finished reading this book is to either find a good Reiki master near you or simply ask the universe for a Reiki Master to attune you so that you will be able to really begin your practice.

Commitment

As with any new practice you want to incorporate into your life, the only way that it will become an integral and important part of your life is if you make a commitment to it. If you want to use the art of healing successfully and integrate it into your everyday life, you need to make space and time every day to practice it.

The most important things in your life should have priority. And what can be more important than bettering yourself in all sorts of ways. Whether you already have a practice of meditating, doing yoga, journaling, or working out, this is another aspect of taking care of yourself in order to be the best version of you today and in the future.

So the first part of committing is deciding how much you want to commit. Although every day is certainly a great ideal, if you do not think that this is a commitment you can actually put on your schedule and achieve, then this is not a promise you will want to make to yourself. You do not want to tell yourself you will do it every day and then beat yourself up if you do not get around to it. Decide how many days a week you want to begin focusing on your practice. You do not need large chunks of time. These do not have to be unmanageable events on your calendar. Perhaps you want to spend 30 minutes three days a week. Find your daily schedule and block out time for it. Perhaps you want to spend five minutes a day, every day. Make sure you know what time exactly those five minutes will occur, or you will not be committing to it.

There is no best schedule for anyone, nor is there any best time of day to work on it. The absolute best schedule for working on your Reiki is at whatever frequency and whatever time is best for you to actually do it. Perhaps you want to begin your day with it, in which case maybe you want to practice Reiki yourself first thing in the morning. Or maybe you have difficulty getting to sleep at night and therefore you could use this focus just before bed. Maybe you need a midday break during a stressful workday and there for a lunchtime routine would work best for you. There is no judgment or preferences outside of what works best for you. In fact, you might very well find that all three are what work best for you.

Prepare

Finally, before you get started with even your very first Reiki session, you want to be physically and mentally prepared. Every single person will be different, so exactly what you may need varies from person to person, however, there are few things everyone can do to best get ready for the journey they are about to embark upon.

You are going to want to be the best mindset that you can put yourself in. This means that in order to stay focused and not get distracted you will want to have eaten a small meal about half an hour before you get started. You do not want to eat anything heavy, as this is more likely to make you sleepy. Nor do you want to eat anything that is especially difficult to digest, as you will very likely be distracted by that. Nor do you want to be especially thirsty throughout your session. You should have some water beforehand, but not so much that you will need to use the restroom frequently throughout. It is advisable to avoid caffeine, as this is going to alter your natural state. Along those same lines, you are not going to want to be under the influence of recreational drugs or alcohol. These will all alter the energy already flowing through you, thereby changing the very thing which you are trying to work on.

It is important to be rested for your session, because you do not want to become so sleepy that you fall asleep during the relaxing Reiki session. It is also important that you use the time before your session to try to clear your mind of any outside distractions. Rather than thinking about what has already happened in your day or what is still left on your to-do list, this is a time to focus on the present and possibly even reflect on why you were at this juncture in the first place, and perhaps what you hope to get out of this journey.

It is very important for your Reiki session that you are comfortable. If you are constantly fidgeting with a pair of pants that digs into your hips, or have your hair tied so tightly that it is giving you a headache, these are all going to be not only major distractions, but also, they are going to alter the energy that you are trying to work with. Some things to consider are what you're wearing, as well as the temperature. Be ready to have layers to add or subtract in order to adjust accordingly to help cool or warm yourself, depending upon what your location is.

If you are working with a Reiki master, you are going to want to ask them if they have any suggestions, recommendations, or rules about how you should prepare beforehand. A lot of practitioners have very specific rules such as: eliminating meat from your diet in the days leading up to your first session, going on a juice cleanse, eliminating alcohol for a few days prior, eliminating smoking from your days leading up to your session, possibly even going on a media diet of avoiding any outside media consumption, and in some cases, spending a good portion of time prior to your session in silence and solitude.

You should also ask what to expect before going into your first session. Most likely the space you will be in will be a quiet, calm, and inviting space. There may or may not be music, white noise, or silence. If you have a preference, it is absolutely appropriate to voice these to your Reiki master, but there is also a good chance they have a reason for their own preference, so feel free to ask them about that. If you will be receiving Reiki from them, you will probably do so while laying down, however, it can also certainly be done sitting or standing. This should happen while you are fully clothed and comfortable in your surroundings. This is going to include them putting their hands on and near your body. However, you should absolutely always feel safe enough to discuss with your Reiki master exactly what you do and do not feel appropriate. Under no circumstances should it hurt or feel uncomfortable to you. If you have any areas of concern, perhaps you have an injury, perhaps you are especially ticklish, or perhaps you certain simply do not want to be touched in a certain spot, this is something you can and should share with them. If they are not receptive to any of this information, you should not practice with them.

To that end, there are also a few things you should do the following your first session, and therefore be prepared for before you even begin. Much like the preparations, these things include many of the same suggestions, but include more reflection. Some Reiki Masters will ask you to do a three, seven, or even twenty-one-day cleanse of many of the aforementioned things such as alcohol, smoking, meat, and media. There will likely be a lot of thoughts and reflections happening, so being prepared with a journal is a good idea. And of course being well-rested, well-hydrated, and well-nourished is an important part of your health, healing, and newly budding Reiki practice.

Chapter 6: History Of Reiki

As you begin to learn and master Reiki, it is a good idea to read about its history. For many years, after all, the practice has had a colorful journey. From its humble beginnings to its current status, Reiki can offer enlightenment. It will also help you understand why it is what it is now. It may be confusing at some points, and you wonder how some aspects of Reiki changed. However, once you have reached the end, you will realize what the practice is all about.

Origins of Reiki

Reiki by itself has a tricky origin. Long before the current healing system came to be, there were already at least four methods being practiced in Japan. One of them, which was known as Reiki Ryoho, was established back in 1914. There was even a book published by its creator,

Matiji Kawakami. Nevertheless, only one person in history would come to make Reiki one of the world's popular healing methods: Dr. Mikao Usui.

Born to a rich clan in 1865, Dr. Usui's early years were all good on his end. His family gave him the resources to have a great education and allowed him to study in a Buddhist monastery where he learned exceptional skills that would benefit him in his lifetime.

Dr. Usui became more interested in medicine, psychology, and theology while studying. Throughout those early years, he had a growing desire to find a way to heal not only himself but also others by using the method that involved laying hands on aching body parts. He wanted to find a healing method that wasn't attached to a specific religion and was available for everyone as well.

It was known that Dr. Usui traveled a lot, studying all types of practices and holding different professions. Then, he became a Buddhist monk and lived in a monastery.

While training, Dr. Usui was on a rediscovery course in a cave at Mt. Kurama. That's where he fasted, prayed, and meditated for 21 days. On the 21st day, he experienced an event like no other: He saw ancient Sanskrit symbols that would guide him toward developing the healing method known as Usui Reiki. While there were other methods that bore the name Reiki, this was the first time in history when it finally had its place in the world.

Sometime after the event, Dr. Usui went to Kyoto to put up his own clinic. This was where he built Usui Reiki. Soon enough, he gained popularity because of this. All of a sudden, the world came to know Reiki. What was once an obscure method became popular.

As Dr. Usui began to gain ground with his practice, he shared his knowledge and taught several students who would later become Reiki masters. His goal was to keep the healing system from being forgotten.

One of Dr. Usui's students, Dr. Chujiro Hayashi, was credited for enhancing the Usui Reiki system by adding hand positions to cover more areas of the body, refining the attunement procedure, and teaching more individuals. He even kept records of the illnesses and symptoms that patients had in order to keep a close eye on how the methods were doing. After that, he made a handbook for practitioners.

Dr. Usui asked Dr. Hayashi to put up his own clinic and teach the Reiki healing system to others. He would later fulfill this request, as well as establish a school.

In the years since Dr. Usui's death, the Usui Reiki system spread far and wide to a point that it has become one of the world's sacred healing systems.

Branches of Reiki in the East and West

As Reiki began to gain popularity, distinct branches in the East and West started to rise as well. For the Eastern branches, everything has obviously been established in Japan first, thanks to Dr. Mikao Usui. Then, after Dr. Chujiro Hayashi learned how the practice worked, he taught Reiki to a lot of students. One of them continued to practice the traditions and decided to be respectful of Usui's original teachings by not making use of the non-Japanese elements previously added to Usui Reiki. This was where Jikiden Reiki came to life.

The practice also came to India. The practitioners in the country integrated the Indian culture to Reiki at the time, such as aura and chakra healing. They also added Hindu deities as part of the practice, along with yoga and Tibet-like elements to make it more distinct than the other types of Reiki known around the world. In this way, the Reiki healing gained a sub-category.

For the Western branches, on the other hand, Reiki began with a woman named Hawayo Takata in 1935. While living in Hawaii, she was ill and needed to undergo surgery. However, Takata was against the latter because she felt that she did not need to go through with it. When she asked her doctor about other possible treatments, Takata was told that someone was practicing Reiki in Tokyo. Even though she was not aware of what it was at the time, she decided to make an appointment with the practitioner who turned out to be Dr. Hayashi.

Hawayo Takata was skeptical about Reiki when she heard about it for the first time. But after going on a few more sessions, she began to feel relaxed. The healing process started sooner than later as well. Takata was so impressed by the fact that she was getting better and better, to the point that she wondered if the practitioners were using secret equipment to conduct the treatment. Over time, though, her doubts melted away when she finally gave in to the wonders of Reiki.

Hawayo Takata felt so much change in her body that, with Dr. Hayashi's help, she started practicing Reiki healing and managed to climb Levels 1 and 2. Then, when she went back to the USA, she continued doing Reiki. It took some time, but Takata eventually became a master and reached Level 3. From there, she opened her own clinic and established the first Western branch, which was also known as Usui Reiki.

Many of her students said that Takata influenced the way Western Reiki works today. After all, based on her experience, she felt that the Japanese method was a bit too complicated and that there were too many things to remember and do. So, she tried to simplify the system by lessening the number of attunements required, omitting some of the traditional systems that were intact at the time, and giving more emphasis on other aspects (such as the symbols) to make the learning process easier for her students.

Since then, the Western branch grew bigger, and more Reiki believers came to master the system, as well as the other additions that came later. At present, many people across the globe understood the Western version better, including the new masters from Japan.

Types of Reiki

As you will no doubt learn, Reiki has different types, so it can be confusing to know which is which. You may find that the Reiki session you are about to try is not like the previous session that you have had the other day, for instance. There may even be techniques that are not taught in the usual way. You might also see symbols that will be marked as non-traditional. do not worry, though, because we will list are the types of Reiki commonly practiced worldwide below.

Usui Reiki

Founded by Mikao Usui, healing is done through Usui Reiki by laying the hands on various body parts. Also classified as the Western Reiki, it is the most typically used type of Reiki in the world. Despite being called as such, this Reiki is also used in Japan.

What makes Usui Reiki useful for many people is that its principles, guidelines, and benefits are more familiar than others. This type has had many additional elements added to it in recent years, so much of the original system is not present in Western Reiki. Then, there was a time when Takata took a little spin on things and simplified the system to make it easier for everyone to understand and follow.

Usui Reiki happens to be the standard type of Reiki. Its healing techniques can be found in Chapters 8 and 9, so they should be clear for you when you practice starts.

Jikiden Reiki

Jikiden Reiki is the opposite of Usui Reiki because it is known as the Eastern Reiki. Unlike the Usui Reiki, Jikiden Reiki's principles and methods are different because they do not have non-Japanese elements like the other healing practices. Established by Chiyoko Yamaguchi, one of Dr. Hayashi's students, this type also keeps the five principles (which you will learn about in Chapter 4) a vital part of the practice. To put it simply, this is what Usui's Reiki system would be like if he was still alive and kept the tradition intact. So, if you are more interested in mastering the original method of healing, Jikiden Reiki is the way to go.

Lightarian Reiki

Lightarian Reiki is a type of Reiki that has been described as a method that can help you accelerate spiritual growth and access a broad range of healing energies. Inspired by the Buddha, Lightarian Reiki also lets you achieve abilities that can be used to help others when healing them. This Reiki practice has been known to help cut the unwanted cords between people as well.

Unlike the other types of Reiki described above, Lightarian Reiki has its own levels or degrees and processes when you try to ascend through them. In truth, it comes with more levels than the Usui Reiki. It even has an institute that will help you go through everything. Lightarian Reiki also requires you to be a licensed practitioner with a few years of experience in practicing other forms of Reiki; that's why it is recommended for seasoned individuals who are ready to take their Reiki skills to a whole new level.

Sekhem or Seichem/Seichim Reiki

Sekhem or Seichem Reiki is a type of Reiki that obtains healing energy from the Egyptian Goddess Akhmet. Classified as a high-vibrational energy healing system, this practice incorporates four elements (earth, air, fire, and water) and ancient symbols with various meanings. This type of Reiki encourages every practitioner to take responsibility for their lives and dig deeper into their souls. It also has a negative energy drain method in which your job is to drain all the negativities that you feel within. After finishing the process, you will feel calmer and have a clearer mind. In other ways, this type of Reiki allows you to look deeper within than you ever thought possible.

Karuna Reiki

Karuna Reiki is a type of Reiki in which the healing energy is more focused in its methods. Developed by William Rand, it makes use of symbols that mean a lot more than they look. They do not use the ones that are traditionally used in Usui Reiki, but they still pack a punch. It is also the type that helps practitioners take the action that they want and has a lot more benefits than other Reiki types discussed here, such as healing the suffering, gentler healing, and many more. If you are ready to take the gentleness to a deeper level, look no further than this method.

Though all the Reiki types mentioned above are different from each other, one thing is sure: all of them continue to develop. Since Dr. Mikao Usui made Reiki healing accessible all over the world with the help of his students, its history indicates that the methods will never be stagnant. It will continue to grow and help others. After all, its source of energy is infinite and cultivated all around us. There are even more Reiki types than the ones listed above, so who knows what the future brings and where it will go next.

Chapter 7: Reiki Attunement

As explained earlier, reiki healing is not taught in the traditional student-master classroom technique. Reiki learning involves the process of attunement, sometimes referred to as initiation.

Reiki attunement, referred to as Reiju in Japanese, is a powerful spiritual experience in which the student's palm, heart, and crown chakras are opened and a special connection is created between the Reiki source and the student. In this process, the Reiki Master channelizes the power of the attunement energies or the Qi into the student.

Moreover, the attunement process is guided by Rei or the Divine Power, and adjustments are automatically made depending on the needs and the capability of the student. Reiki spiritual beings including guides attend this initiation process offering help in its implementation.

Many students have reported mystical experiences during the attunement in the form of personal messages, past life experiences, healings, and visions. The attunement also helps in improving the student's psychic sensitivities. Many people have reported other-worldly experiences such as the opening of their third eye and significantly improved intuitive abilities.

Once students complete an attunement, they will have access to Reiki energy source throughout their lives. The effect of the attunement does not wear off nor will you lose it. However, additional attunements are beneficial in many ways including refinement and increased strength of the Reiki energy that the student is channeling, increased psychic abilities, improved self-healing, clarity of mind, and an increased level of consciousness.

Pre-Attunement Preparations

Before the period of attunement, it is good to follow a process of purification to enable the energies to work more efficiently than otherwise. Although this preparation period is not mandatory, many Reiki masters recommend it. Here are some pointers to becoming prepared to receive Reiki energy:

• Avoid meats, fish, and all other non-vegetarian foods for three days before the attunement. These foods are known to increase the sluggishness in our body and mind throwing it out of balance.

• It is best to try juice or water fasting for a day before D-day, especially if you already have experience with fasting and being vegetarian

• Reduce or minimize the use of caffeinated drinks like coffee and tea. Caffeine creates imbalances in the endocrine and nervous systems. On the day of the attunement, you must stay away from coffee.

- Avoid alcohol completely, if possible, and certainly for three days before the attunement day

- Avoid the intake of sweets and chocolates completely

- Cut back on smoking, and if possible, it is best to give it up entirely. On the day of the attunement, you must necessarily give up smoking completely

- For a week before the decided day, try and meditate for an hour daily. Even if you are not used to meditation, spend some me-time doing nothing but being with yourself and your thoughts. You can go for long walks in the midst of nature. Avoid intense physical activity too.

- Reduce TV watching, reading newspapers, and listening to the radio. Instead, focus on your feelings, thoughts, and sensations from within and around you. Contemplate on the senses and emotions

- Let go of all negative emotions including anger, hate, jealousy, fear, worries, anxiety, etc. and let them be taken up and consumed by the light. Focus a sacred aura around you.

Reiki attunement is the first level of Reiki learning. Self-Reiki is the ultimate goal of this first level. It encourages students to practice the healing techniques of Reiki on themselves to clear obstacles and energy blockages in their body and mind. Once a student has mastered the first level of self-Reiki, then he or she can move on to the second and third levels.

The second level teaches students to practice Reiki techniques on others. Additionally, it prepares students to expand their energy openings. Students also receive Reiki symbols and attunement into the second level. The symbols (discussed in detail in Chapter 3) help practitioners connect more deeply with the universal energy (or Ki) than before. The second level also teaches you how to provide distance Reiki and help people across time and distance boundaries.

The third level is the master level in which students train to become Reiki masters wherein they can attune new Reiki practitioners and help them receive Ki. Some people complete this level successfully and yet are not comfortable giving in practicing attunement on others.

Therefore, this Reiki level is clearly distinguished from the master level in which the practitioner not only completes the third level successfully including receiving symbols and attunement but also is comfortable with initiating new Reiki practitioners into the sacred realm as well as practicing Reiki healing techniques on other people.

Thus, becoming a Reiki Master calls for a deep level of continued commitment to

Reiki practice. Many masters believe that a considerable time must pass after learning and mastering the second level before attempting to try the third level.

Chapter 8: What Is Reiki?

The word Reiki comes from two Japanese words Rei & Ki, the Japanese Kanji ideograms have many levels of meanings.

Reiki is "Spiritually Guided Life Force Energy"

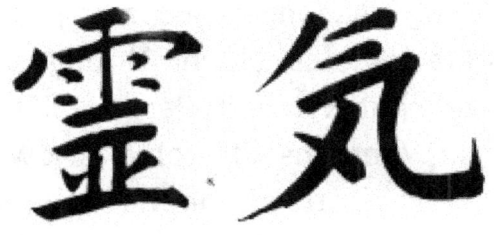

REI: Spiritual Wisdom, KI: Life Force Energy

Higher Power, Universal

REI means Universal and an esoteric meaning is supernatural knowledge or spiritual consciousness. It is the wisdom that comes from God or the higher self.

This is the God consciousness, which all knows. It understands each person completely. It knows the cause of all problems and difficulties and knows what to do to heal them.

KI means the same as Chi in Chinese, Prana in Sanskriti, Ti or Ki in Hawaiian. It has also been called odic force, organ and bioplasma. Rei is the universal life force, the non-physical energy that animates all living things. As long as something is alive, it has life force circulating through it and surrounding it. When it dies, the life force departs. When the life force is low or if there is a restriction in its flow, living beings are more vulnerable to stickiness. The life force plays an important role in everything that we do. Besides animating the body, it is also the primary energy of our emotions, thoughts and spiritual life.

It is the God consciousness called REI that guides the universal life force called Ki in the practice we call Reiki, Reiki can be defined as spiritually guided energy.

Reiki guides itself with its own wisdom. This practitioner doesn't decide what to heal and can't direct Reiki with his intention. The practitioner is not the doer/healer; the practitioner is only a channel through which Reiki flows. Reiki flows more freely when the practitioner can put his ego and mind out of the way (meditation during the treatment helps), leaving everything to Reiki, surrendering to Reiki.

As long as the practitioner is a true channel (the mind/ego are not involved), he is protected from taking, karma and sickness from the patients. If the practitioner tricks to be the healer, to take away pain/sickness with his mind, he might start doing psychic healing instead of Reiki, and take on himself the sickness or karma of the patient.

Because Reiki is guided by God consciousness, it can never harm, it knows what the person needs and will adjust itself to create the effect that is appropriate from them.

Because Reiki is channeled healing, the practitioner doesn't use his own energies and his energies don't get depleted during a treatment. In fact, giving a treatment increases one's energy since Reiki consciousness considered both the practitioner and patient to be in need of healing, so both receive a treatment.

— Reiki is not

Religious. Reiki is totally nondenominational. You can practice any religion or none and still use and benefit from Reiki. People of all faiths ad beliefs are Reiki practitioners.

Massage or Reflexology.

A form of psychic healing.

A form of min control wishful thinking or hypnosis.

Meditation technique.

Chapter 9: History Of Reiki

The Reiki strategy for recuperating was established on the disclosure and comprehension of the body's vitality framework. Reiki Practitioners endeavor to improve wellbeing and personal satisfaction by offering Reiki vitality and reestablishing harmony. Reiki is utilized in self-care, for consideration of one's family, and is offered in private practive and in emergency clinics and restorative settings as an aide and steady treatment to health and conventional medicinal consideration. The type of Reiki that numerous individuals practice today, Usui Reiki, has been being used for more than one hundred years.

The Founder of Reiki

The historical backdrop of Usui Reiki starts with its organizer, Dr. Mikao Usui. Now and again called the Usui Sensei, Dr. Mikao

Usui was destined to a well off Buddhist family in 1865. Dr. Usui's family had the option to give their child balanced instruction for the time. As a tyke, Dr. Usui examined in a Buddhist religious community where he was shown hand to hand fighting, swordsmanship, and the Japanese type of Chi Kung, known as Kiko.

All through his training, Dr. Usui had an enthusiasm for drug, brain research and religious philosophy. It was this intrigue incited him to look for an approach to recuperate himself as well as other people utilizing the laying on of hands. It was his longing to discover a technique for recuperating that was unattached to a particular religion and religious conviction, so his framework would be available to everybody.

Dr. Usui voyaged a lot during his lifetime. He concentrated mending frameworks of various types and held various callings including journalist, secretary, teacher, community worker and watchman. At long last, he turned into a Buddhist cleric/priest and lived in a religious community.

Otherworldly Awakening and Development of Reiki

At some point during his long stretches of preparing in the religious community, Dr. Usui went to his very own preparation rediscovery course in a cavern on Mount Kurama. For 21 days, Dr. Usui fasted, contemplated and implored. Moreover, on the morning of the twenty-first day, Dr. Usui encountered an occasion that would change his life for eternity. He saw old Sanskrit images that helped him build up the arrangement of recuperating he had been attempting to design. Usui Reiki was conceived.

After his otherworldly arousing on Mount Kurama, Dr. Usui built up a facility for recuperating and educating in Kyoto. As the act of Usui Reiki was spreading, Dr. Usui ended up known for his recuperating practice.

Other commendable Development about Reiki

Hands on mending has been logically demonstrated to be viable in quickening recuperating

A Reiki treatment bolsters the entire individual including body, feelings, brain and soul making numerous helpful impacts

On a physical level Reiki enables reduction to torment, quickens the mending time of bones and wounds, loosens up muscles and decreases the tissue inclusion of consumes and wounds. It is conceivable to lessen the negative symptoms of medicines, for example, chemotherapy and radiation. Colds, flus, honey bee stings, coronary illness - numerous physical conditions can be treated with Reiki.

On a psychological and passionate level uneasiness is diminished, a feeling of prosperity expanded and another degree of unwinding felt. At this level of profound unwinding a rebalancing of energies happens and the common mending capacity of the body is improved

On a spiritual level, customers have expressed that they feel reawakened and restored after a full-body session

How is a Reiki treatment given?

A run of the mill Reiki treatment will see the customer lying full dressed on a back rub table. It is additionally conceivable to give a Reiki treatment to a customer sitting or standing. The professional places his of her hands on or close to the customer's body in a progression of hand positions from the head to the feet that are held for somewhere in the range of 2 to 10 mins, contingent upon how much time is required at each hand arrangement. The treatment will commonly last somewhere in the range of 45 mins to an hour and may incorporate input acquired by the expert during the treatment. A customer may profit to their professional for a fortnightly reason for some time or may locate that one session gives all the vital advantages. Reiki 2 experts are able to give separation mending meaning you could be anyplace on the planet and get recuperating from your professional.

What does a Reiki treatment feel like?

Everybody will have a somewhat extraordinary encounter anyway regularly individuals feel an a lot further feeling of unwinding. By and by I feel a stunning sparkling brilliance or vitality traveling through my body, here and there in floods and it will move through me and surrounding me. Others will see dreams, or feel like they are drifting over their body. Where the specialist feels blockages in a customer's vitality (and will invest time clearing that blockage) the customer may feel an underlying largeness however then a discharge and stream of vitality. It isn't unordinary for customers to encounter a passionate discharge as enthusiastic disturbance is brought to the surface and discharged.

Reiki is likewise a profound practice that develops genuine feelings of serenity, improves our wellbeing and essentialness, and advances mental prosperity. Every day self-Reiki medications are a solicitation to health: the establishment of thinking about ourselves and advancing parity and wellbeing on all levels. Reiki is the blessing that continues giving.

The word Reiki implies soul vitality or the vitality of the Universe, which is found in every single living thing, plants and creatures notwithstanding. As individuals, we are altogether brought into the world with Reiki; an attunement or reiju** is everything necessary to enable us to actuate or stir this capacity and recall all that we are able to do.

The training started with Mikao Usui in Japan back in the mid 1920s. Usui's involvement of illumination and deep rooted profound practice drove him to build up the recuperating technique we presently know as Reiki. He created Reiki as a profound practice to develop significant serenity in this way advancing wellbeing and prosperity. Usui Sensei skilled us with the Reiki statutes as devices for mental prosperity and profound development.

** Reiki is certainly not a substitute for medicinal, mental or other social insurance medications.

** A Reiki attunement or reiju is a delicate procedure or strengthening guided by the Reiki Master instructor to enable the understudy to open to, reconnect and line up with, the vitality of the universe and the mending limit that is as of now inside them.

The Reiki strategy for recuperating was established on the disclosure and comprehension of the body's vitality framework. Reiki Practitioners endeavor to improve wellbeing and personal satisfaction by offering Reiki vitality and reestablishing harmony. Reiki is utilized in self-care, for consideration of one's family, and is offered in private practive and in emergency clinics and therapeutic settings as an assistant and steady treatment to wellbeing and customary medicinal consideration. The type of Reiki that numerous individuals practice today, Usui Reiki, has been being used for more than one hundred years.

The historical backdrop of Usui Reiki starts with its originator, Dr. Mikao Usui. Once in a while called the Usui Sensei, Dr. Mikao Usui was destined to a well off Buddhist family in 1865. Dr. Usui's family had the option to give their child balanced instruction for the time. As a youngster, Dr. Usui contemplated in a Buddhist religious community where he was shown hand to hand fighting, swordsmanship, and the Japanese type of Chi Kung, known as Kiko.

All through his training, Dr. Usui had an enthusiasm for prescription, brain science and religious philosophy. It was this intrigue incited him to look for an approach to mend himself as well as other people utilizing the laying on of hands. It was his craving to discover a strategy for mending that was unattached to a particular religion and religious conviction, with the goal that his framework would be available to everybody.

Dr. Usui voyaged a lot during his lifetime. He concentrated mending frameworks of numerous kinds and held various callings including columnist, secretary, preacher, community worker and watchman. At long last, he turned into a Buddhist minister/priest and lived in a religious community.

At some point during his long stretches of preparing in the religious community, Dr.

Usui went to his very own preparation rediscovery course in a cavern on Mount Kurama. For 21 days, Dr. Usui fasted, thought and supplicated. And on the morning of the twenty-first day, it happened that Dr. Usui encountered an occasion that would change his life for eternity. He saw antiquated Sanskrit images that helped him build up the arrangement of mending he had been attempting to imagine. Usui Reiki was conceived.

After his profound arousing on Mount Kurama, Dr. Usui built up a facility for mending and instructing in Kyoto. As the act of Usui Reiki was spreading, Dr. Usui ended up known for his mending practice.

In the mid 1990s there were disclosures of Usui's unique Reiki lessons. The commemoration of Usui was found by western instructors and many people from Reiki's missing connections were revealed. Disclosures incorporated the revelation of a living Reiki custom in Japan, with extra strategies as instructed by the Reiki Gakkai (Reiki Learning Society). Some of Usui's notes and manuals were likewise shared and this prompted more noteworthy disclosures which were later made all the more by and large accessible. Western Reiki instructors increased new data seeing the framework as it had been educated in Japan and this was sorted out with set up frameworks of Reiki in the West.

Usui's Students

On first September 1923, the devasting Kanto tremor stuck Tokyo and encompassing regions. A large portion of the focal piece of Tokyo was leveled and completely pulverized by flame. More than 140,000 individuals were murdered. In one case, 40,000 individuals were burned when a flame tornado cleared over the open territory where they had looked for wellbeing. Tragically the quake struck at late morning, exactly when individuals' charcoal flame broils were set to prepare lunch. 3,000,000 homes were pulverized, leaving endless destitute. More than 50,000 individuals endured genuine wounds. The open water and sewage frameworks were obliterated and it took a very long time for re-working to happen.

In light of this disaster, Usui and his understudies offered Reiki to incalculable unfortunate casualties. His facility turned out to be too little to even consider handling the crowds of patients, so in February 1924, he manufactured another center in Nakano, outside Tokyo. His notoriety spread rapidly all through Japan and he started accepting solicitations from everywhere throughout the nation to come and show his recuperating techniques. Usui was granted a Kun San To from the Emperor, which is a high grant (much like a privileged doctorate), given to the individuals who had done respectable work. His acclaim before long spread all through the district also, numerous noticeable healers and doctors started mentioning lessons from him.

Usui rapidly turned out to be occupied as solicitations for instructing Reiki kept on developing. He voyaged broadly all through Japan which was not a simple endeavor back then, to instruct and give Reiki attunements. This began to negatively affect his wellbeing and he started encountering smaller than expected strokes from pressure. On ninth March, 1926, while in Fukuyama, Usui kicked the bucket of a lethal stroke. He was 62 years of age.

It is said that Usui instructed Reiki to a little more than 2000 individuals and out of these understudies a few sources state he prepared 22 to educator level(Shinpiden). Huge numbers of these understudies started their very own centers and established Reiki schools and social orders. Not these educator level understudies are known outside of Japan.

By the 1940s there were around 40 Reiki schools spread all over Japan. The vast majority of these schools showed the strategy for Reiki that Usui had created.

Dr Chujiro Hayashi

The ancestry of most of Western Reiki experts springs from Chuijro Hayashi. Hayashi read with Mikao Usui for somewhere in the range of ten months preceding Usui's passing. He is accepted to have changed a portion of the strategies of Usui.

Chuijro Hayashi was conceived in 1879. At some point in 1925 Chuijro Hayashi met Usui. Chuijro had ascended to be an authority in the Imperial Navy and had prepared in Western and Chinese Medicine. In June of 1925, Hayashi got his instructor's preparation in Usui's framework. A few sources state that Chuijro Hayashi was a Methodist Christian, a reality affirmed one of his Shoden/Okudent understudies,

Mrs.Yamaguchi. Different sources state that he was a Soto Zen specialist who used the acts of Shinto. For all we know, he may have been both as this would be flawlessly as per Japanese ways to deal with religion. As a Christian, Hayashi would have taken in the rearranged type of Reiki.

Before his demise on tenth May 1940 Hayashi adjusted 13 understudies to the educator level, incorporating Hawayo Takata in 1938.

Mrs Takata - Usui Shiki Ryoh

Hawayo Kawamura (her original last name), was brought into the world 25th December 1900 in Hanamaula, Kauai, Hawaii. On the tenth March 1917 she wedded her significant other, Saichi Takata. They had two little girls, one named Alice Takata-Furumoto, who later had a little girl named Phyllis Furumoto.

It is because of Mrs Takata that Reiki is outstanding and wide-spread all through the world. Mrs. Takata officially brought

Reiki to terrain America in the start of the 1970s and during a multi year time frame, encouraged 22 Western understudies to the instructor level. Her style of Reiki created from what she was educated by Dr Hayashi.

It was following the demise of her significant other in 1930 and afterward her sister in 1935 that Hawayo Takata chose to go to Japan to visit her folks. Because of diligent work to help her family and sadness, Takata's wellbeing had started to endure. She was booked to have an activity in Japan to help settle her medical issues. Just before the activity she heard the voice of her dead spouse, saying that the activity was a bit much and that there was another way. This provoked her to talk with her primary care physician about elective medicines and he alluded her on to Hayashi's Reiki Clinic.]Hawayo Takata gotten day by day medications at this facility for a time of four months and during this time her manifestations totally subsided.

This drove Hawayo Takata to take Reiki One preparing (Shoden) with Hayashi on tenth December 1935. She examined the principal level with him for barely one year. In 1937, Mrs. Takata got the subsequent level, Okuden. Soon after this, she came back to Hawaii. Half a month later, Hayashi visited Mrs. Takata with his little girl and remained until February 1938. During this time Hayashi authoritatively made Mrs. Takata a Reiki educator.

Somewhere in the range of 1940 and 1970, Mrs. Takata ran a few Reiki centers and showed numerous classes in Hawaii. In 1973 she showed her five star in the United States itself. In December of 1980 Mrs. Takata kicked the bucket. Much appreciation and affirmation is perceived for Mrs. Takata in empowering Reiki to spread all through the world. Without her, the arrangement of Reiki may have right up 'til the present time stayed obscure but to a chosen few in Japan.

Dr Usui's Original Reiki Teachings

The more profound otherworldly practices and procedures of the Japanese conventions, notwithstanding, have stayed behind Japan's shut Reiki society. The first Reiki of Mikao Usui still thrives in Japan yet is impressively unique practically speaking. Outside of Japan there are just three authourised educators of the pre-1922 framework – one of whom is an individual from The Reiki Guild.

Chapter 10: How Reiki Began: The History

The Plight of Usui Reiki

The Reiki healing technique was established when people began to understand the mechanism of energy in the body.

Reiki Practitioners endeavor to improve wellbeing and personal satisfaction by offering Reiki energy and balance restoration.

Reiki is utilized in self-care, for the care of one's family, and is offered in private practice and in emergency clinics and therapeutic settings as an assistant and strong treatment to health and conventional medicinal consideration.

The type of Reiki that numerous individuals practice today, Usui Reiki, has been being used for more than one hundred years.

The historical backdrop of Usui Reiki starts with its organizer, Dr. Mikao Usui. Popularly nicknamed the Usui Sensei, Dr. Mikao Usui was destined to a well off Buddhist family in 1865. Dr. Usui's family had the option to give their child balanced training for the time. As a youngster, Dr. Usui examined in a Buddhist religious community where he was shown combative techniques, swordsmanship, and the Japanese type of Chi Kung, known as Kiko.

All through his instruction, Dr. Usui had an enthusiasm for medication, brain science and philosophy. It was this intrigue that incited him to look for an approach to self-healing as well as other people utilizing the laying on of hands. It was his longing to discover a technique for healing that was unattached to a particular religion and strict conviction. Also, he wanted a framework that would be available to everybody.

Dr. Usui voyaged a lot during his lifetime. He read a lot about healing techniques of numerous kinds and held various callings including correspondent, secretary, preacher, community worker and gatekeeper. At long last, he turned into a Buddhist cleric/priest and lived in a monastery.

At some point during his long periods of preparing in the cloister, Dr. Usui went to his very own preparation rediscovery course in a cavern on Mount Kurama. For 21 days, Dr. Usui fasted, prayed and reflected. On the morning of the twenty-first day, Dr. Usui encountered an occasion that would change his life until the end of time. He saw old Sanskrit images that helped him build up the exact healing system he had been imagining. Usui Reiki was conceived.

After his spiritual rebirth on Mount Kurama, Dr. Usui built up a facility for healing and instructing in Kyoto. As the act of Usui Reiki was spreading, Dr. Usui ended up known for his healing practice.

The Development and Spread of Reiki Meditation

Mikao Usui established his first Reiki center and school in Tokyo in 1922. Before his demise, Dr. Usui instructed a few Reiki bosses to guarantee that his self-healing method would not be overlooked. Among them was Dr. Chujiro Hayashi, a previous maritime official who set up a Reiki center in Tokyo.

Dr. Hayashi is credited with further building up the Usui arrangement of Reiki by adding hand positions so that the healing process can cover the whole body. Dr. Hayashi additionally changed and refined the attunement procedure. Utilizing his improved framework, Dr. Hayashi taught a few more Reiki Masters, including a lady named Hawayo Takata. Mrs. Takata was a Japanese-American lady who initially went to Dr. Hayashi for personal healing. After learning the frameworks herself, Mrs. Takata took Reiki home to the United States.

Hawayo Takata was in Tokyo in 1935. Mrs. Takata was exceptionally sick and needing a medical procedure. But she knew, through intuition, that she didn't require surgery to recuperate. She spoke with her primary care physician about elective medicines for her condition, she was told about the Reiki expert around the local area. Mrs. Takata had never known about Reiki, yet she made an arrangement, despite the fact that she was unsure of the outcome. After the first meeting with Dr. Hayashi, Mrs. Takata saw Dr. Hayashi once a day. She saw the sessions as unwinding and wonderful and, eventually, recuperating.

As time passed, Mrs. Takata learned Reiki One and Reiki Two. At the point when she came back to the United States, Mrs. Takata kept on rehearsing Reiki and in the end turned into a Reiki Master. Quite a bit of this occurred close to the start of World War II.

Mrs. Takata needed to spread her arrangement of recuperating to other people. She made changes to her Reiki practice, at that point utilized Reiki to help heal others in the United States.

Prior to his death, Dr. Hayashi figured out how to confer all of Dr. Usui's lessons onto Mrs. Takata. She kept on rehearsing Reiki for a long time. Before Mrs. Takata's death, she had taught and made attunements for 22 Reiki masters.

Today, individuals who practice Reiki utilize the techniques created by Dr. Usui, the author of Usui Reiki. The uniqueness of Reiki is that professionals can use Reiki to help treat themselves for their own health and improved prosperity. Truth be told, using Reiki personally is a key criterion for offering the practice to other people. Present day Reiki experts can offer the Reiki vitality to others through delicate static light weight touch utilizing the particular customary Reiki hand positions and even over distant people: this is similar to faith prayers. Reiki can be used together with numerous restorative treatments and customary prescription and can be utilized to help aid the potential treatment of individuals experiencing pains, ailment, malady and a lot more.

Contemporary Reiki is ending up increasingly mainstream over the long haul, and the lineage of Reiki experts is developing each day. With the arrival of Usui Reiki, numerous individuals are utilizing this conventional hands on treatment to heal themselves as well as other people.

Chapter 11: History Of Reiki

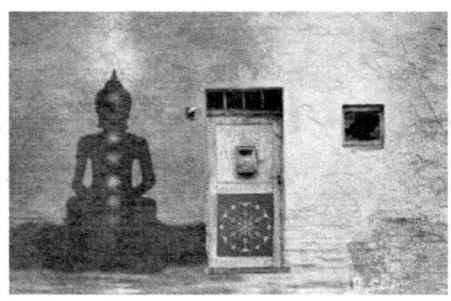

Reiki in Japanese became diluted because of its passage from one generation to another through word of mouth. The passage of the information made the name of this powerful art disappear. So many people practicing this powerful art believe that Japanese is not the original home of Reiki. They believe Reiki was first used by the Indian Buddha, and then it was moved down to Jesus of the Christian religion.

There is a specific timeframe that shows when Reiki was born. The history of the time of the birth of Reiki is speculative. No proof has been found to show when the living things learned how to get this universal force of life and put it into practice to heal themselves and the others. Some people have even looked at the very old times, but still, they did not get to know when Reiki started.

The real knowledge of when Reiki came into being is in reiki's rediscovery. This powerful art was discovered again by a monk known as Dr. Mikao Usui. There is real proof of the timeframe in which he discovered this art. The Reiki was rediscovered in the ninetieth century by Dr Mikao Usui. Despite the rediscovery of the powerful force by the monk, after his death apart from the tomb, he was buried in Tokyo; there has been limited material evidence that points out his work and accomplishments during his lifetime.

When you look at different records of the history of Reiki, you will realize that Dr. Mikao Usui was a Christian monk who was also a lecturer at Do shisha University that is located in Tokyo.

Doctor Mikao Usui as much as he believed in the universal super force that heals, he denied the fact walking on water by Jesus Christ, raising the dead, healing the blind, healing the lame, turning water into wine and several other miracles that Jesus performed were beyond his understanding and capabilities. His declaration of these in capabilities was confirmed when he answered a question from the student who asked him if he believed in Christianity and could perform all the miracles that Jesus did.

The history continues to say that after Dr. Mikao Usui answering the student's question by saying he had no capabilities that Jesus had, he resigned from his job and developed another course in search of the power to heal and perform miracles as

Jesus had done. The history is very doubtful, especially when it says that Dr Mikao Usui began searching for the secrets of Jesus Christ on how he performed his miracles at the University of Chicago.

The Reiki Master William Rand came to rescue of Dr. Mikao Usui's repetition and disapproved of the history of the devaluation of their rediscovery master going to the University of Chicago in search of knowledge on how Jesus performed miracles so that he can perform them in the same way.

Reiki Master William proved that there is single evidence that proofs Dr. Mikao Usui lectured at Doshia University in Tokyo. The western society has constantly changed the history of the master of the rediscovery of Reiki to suit them, but there are so many gaps left unfilled that put so many unanswered questions in the truth of this history of the legend.

Life of Dr. Mikao Usui

The generation that Dr. Mikao was born in was in the Zen Buddhism religion practice. They had been practicing it for eleven generations down the line when Dr Usui was born. During the youthful stage of Doctor Mikao Usui, the fascination of all things in the western engulfed him, but unfortunately, he never satisfied them because he did not travel anywhere further than Japan. After finishing his school, he joined allopathic medicine with other western physicians. His spiritual revelation came when he got sick from a cholera outbreak that had massively attacked Tokyo at large and was at the verge of dying.

He later joined a monastery, and after many years of studying, he discovered the references for a very different type of healing. He went further and discovered that there were ways of how one can learn about this healing energy and be able to use it. Some symbols and formulas showed how one could use the palms of the hand to heal using this energy. Despite Usui finding this power and the ways of using it, he still didn't have any knowledge of what they meant and how he was going to start using them. For this fact, he decides to go deep into meditation and find the answers to this puzzle that he had found. It needed a final touch so that the kit could go into use.

Doctor Usui decided to take a leave from the monastery after some meditation and went to the holy mountain to get the interpretation of the unique energy he had discovered so that it can be in use. On the mountain, he collected twenty-one small stones that he used during his meditation while reading the sacred scriptures called the sutras for 21 days. Each day on the mountain that he meditated, he threw away a stone to mark it ending as he also sang.

On his last day, he asked God for a miracle through a sign. He needed to know if all his meditation had gone through and a sign of the light was all he wanted from God. God seemingly answered his prayer as a very bright light came from the sky and hit him hard on the forehead. Usui fainted, and during this time, his unconscious spirit saw the same symbols and the sutras that he had seen earlier.

This revelation was that entire doctor Usui needed. He now had proof and full knowledge that this old power of healing existed and was used by Buddha and Jesus. After sometimes on the mountain for the recovery of his consciousness fully, he started going down the mountain, but he hit his toe hard on the rock that I was so painful and bled much. Usui placed his hand on the toe, and the pain subsided and left the toe while the bleeding miraculously stopped.

On his way, Usui went to a village to eat for he was hungry after fasting for the 21 days. The surprising thing is that he ate comfortably without any complications whatsoever, but the waitress that served him had a very painful toothache. Doctor Usui requested to look at that tooth then he placed his hands on her swollen face, and the pain left, and the swelling eased down. After Usui getting enough rest, he continued with his journey back to the monastery. On reaching there, his friend Abbot was in bad shape because of arthritis. Usui was able to place his hands on him, and indeed, Abbot was healed.

All the deeds of Doctor Usui right from the first one to the last one at the monastery were called the four miracles. Doctor Usui's friend being among the witnesses and beneficiary of this gift advice the monk to go to the Kyoto villages ad be able to exercise this gift in healing. He also reminded the doctor Usui that not only is it important to heal the physical body, but it is also important to heal the soul and the mind at large.

After healing and helping the beggars in Kyoto, Usui left, and seven years later, the beggars went back to him, claiming that begging was easier than working. He immediately knew there was something, but since he had forgotten the ritual; he had to do it afresh by going into meditation again. This led to the discovery of the five principles of Reiki. After this, Usui lived healing people using Reiki and teaching them how to use Reiki. He made sure that Reiki was not to be divided by the religious beliefs of different religions or the cultures of different people. Reiki is being used by everyone around the world up to today, making it a universal force of life.

Dr. Mikao Usui died in the year 1930 after initiating all his nineteen students into masters or teachers and after receiving a doctorate from the emperor in appreciation and recognition of his good work. Doctor Usui was succeeded by Chujiro Hayashi after his death. Doctor Hayashi, a qualified physician from a high-class family and a retired commander, continued the good works of Doctor Usui.

He decided to build a healing clinic in Tokyo called Shina No Macha where his students healed people using Reiki. The students also visited the homes of the sick who had no capabilities in traveling. Doctor Chujiro Hayashi wrote so much about the treatments and the required diets by people receiving this treatment. He advanced Reiki to another level when he discovered the advantages of healing the whole body and channeling the energies to the right place if you used the full body treatment.

The application of the full body treatment was aimed at removing the toxins in the body. Both the physical and emotional blocks were to be removed if this treatment was to be administered. A situation arose whereby a lady named Taketa fell sick after the demise of her husband's death. The disease was so bad that it reached a state of surgery. The surgery was to be done on the gall bladder. Unfortunately, she also had a respiratory complication that if any pain relievers were to be used on her during the surgery, her chances of survival were minimal. During her sickness and the pain from the death of her husband, her sister died and added another pain to her ailing soul. She traveled to Tokyo to take the bereaving news to her parents.

In the year 1937, she went back to her husband's home town and started her Reiki clinic which was visited by doctor Hayashi in 1938 February when he informed her of being the successor. The war in America came in 1940, but since doctor Hayashi was a peaceful man and did not want to indulge himself in it, he applied his wisdom, and for the preservation of his honor he decided that he will let the leadership go to another person. In Hawaii, one-morning madam Takata visualized doctor Hayashi at her bed foot and decided to go to Japan.

When she arrived, doctor Hayashi talked to her about his plans of dying and they talked a lot planning the future.

After Doctor Chujiro Hayashi seeing the satisfactory results in the Reiki healing and his accomplishments, he summoned all his students and before they appointed madam Taketa as his successor in being the master of Reiki. She was to be the third after Doctor Usui and Doctor Hayashi. After putting things in order by choosing his successor, the grandmaster Hayashi lay down and died. After his death, Madam went back to her clinic in Hawaii and continued with the healing.

The history of Reiki changed when madam Taketa decided to universalize it. She knew it would be very hard for the westerners to accept Reiki stood the chances of being lost again. So she came up with a plan to preserve Reiki by training twenty-two students before she joined her ancestors on December 1980. She made sure before her death that there was a successor to keep reiki's power in progress. The successors of Madam Takata were her granddaughter Phyllis Lei Furumoto and Barbara Weber. The two successors worked together for a year then everyone went their separate way to work. Doctor Barbara weber returned to the western and formed the famous American Reiki Centre (A.I.R.A) while Phyllis Furumoto formed the Reiki Alliance.

Conclusively, the universal force of life, Reiki, is one only it is not divided into different religions or cultures. This super non-physical gift given to us freely is very effective right from the time it was discovered lifting any doubt of it not working.

Chapter 12: Principles Of Reiki

Practice

Reiki is made up of five guiding principles, or Ideals. Using the principles helps us create greater self-empowerment and puts healing into our own hands. Since the original Ideals can be difficult to understand, modern Reiki masters have reworded the principles to make them more "user-friendly." Put into layman's terms, the principles, or Ideals, of Reiki, can be summed up as:

I release angry thoughts and feelings.

I release thoughts of worry.

I am grateful for my many blessings.

I practice expanding my consciousness.

I'm gentle with all beings, including myself.

When we recite these principles, we find ourselves more at peace and empowered to create or change our lives as we choose. Having a phrasing of the Ideals that are easier to understand helps us better understand them, so you can internalize them and evoke them in your Reiki practice. Below is a way to use the principles in everyday life to help with a Reiki practice.

- Recite the first principle out loud to release thoughts and feelings. This can also be recited silently without speaking.

- Think about what has created anger in your life that day, or the previous day. Although most events that cause anger are from outside sources, the anger lives WITHIN us, not WITHOUT. You should recognize that although the event itself was from an outside source, the emotional impact came from the event because we are harboring negative energy inside of us. Then think back to a previous time you were angry and try to find an event that is like the current situation you face. Call upon your Reiki guides, angels, or spirits to help you let go of that anger. As you focus on letting go of the anger, take a couple of deep breaths to re-center and focus yourself. On each exhale, imagine the anger being released from your body and your chi.

• Do the same exercise for the releasing of worry, step two. Think about what is worrying you and connect it to past thoughts of worry. Realize that the worry lives inside of us, not without. The events and situations we are worried about would not bother us if the worry did not already live inside in our minds. Ask your spiritual guides and healers to help you release the worry, taking deep breaths to physically exhale the worry from your body. When you feel your burden lightened, proceed to the next step.

• Think or say out loud that you are grateful for your many blessings. Name, visualize, and feel grateful for each blessing in your life, which might be a person (spouse, child, parents, friends), an object (i.e., feeling grateful to have a home in which to live, or a car to take you to work), or a situation (getting a new job, moving to a new home, etc.). As you visualize your blessings, take deep breaths and allow your heart to expand with gratitude.

- The next step is to think or say the next principle, which is practicing expanding consciousness. Visualize or acknowledge these circumstances that helped expand your consciousness for that day. It might be a meditation or yoga practice, meditating on the Reiki principles, feeling grateful, or even taking a relaxing walk through the woods or on the beach.

- The last principle may be one of the most important to think or say out loud, as it helps us focus on being kind not only to ourselves but to others. We as humans tend to focus on our negative aspects and traits without celebrating what is beautiful about ourselves. Being kind to ourselves can help us open our hearts to being kind to others. Meditate on the times during the day you were not kind to yourself or someone else. Ask your guides to help you release the anxiety of self-beratement and the regret of treating someone unkindly. Inhale light and love, and exhale the negative, heavy energy that you feel.

There is no right or wrong way to study the principles and invoke them in our lives. It is a work in progress that manifests itself differently each day according to our emotions. Practicing the principles of Ideals of Reiki helps us create great peace and balance in our lives, which extends to the lives of others as well.

Chapter 13: Reiki Clothing

Is it possible to acquire the benefits of Reiki without actually practicing it? Is there any other way the energy of Reiki can be communicated? Is there a way to effectively channel the energy of Reiki to others?

Many Reiki healers were involved in various experiments to see if it was possible to impart the healing power others by different means. Thanks to those millions of experiments, now we know various ways in which Reiki can be channeled to others. The most popular way in which energy can be obtained is from Reiki infused clothing.

What is Reiki Clothing?

Reiki clothing refers to clothing that is wholly infused with Reiki energy by an efficient Reiki healer. After a short meditation session, the clothes are infused with Reiki energy. This attire imparts the Reiki energy to those who wear it and surrounds the person with the power of Reiki. Wearing Reiki clothing has a good deal of benefits and you will feel the impact of the Reiki clothing when you switch back to your regular outfit. That is when you will realize the immense transition you went through in all three dimensions of your life - your mind, body and soul.

When can Reiki Clothing be worn?

Reiki clothing holding such great energy can be worn anytime of the day. It can be worn through the day when you are most active going about your daily chores; this way you will be able to carry out your tasks with ease and without your energy being drained. You can also wear this clothing when you go to bed.

This is the time when your body is in recharge mode and if you wear Reiki clothes while sleeping, it will greatly assist the rejuvenation process. You can wear it during celebrations or gatherings to add more radiance to yourself. Reiki clothes are also ideal to wear during any religious ceremonies; the energy would help you connect deep with the superior being.

What materials can be used to make Reiki Clothes?

Reiki clothes are made using different types of cloth, but what really matters is the energy charged into the clothing. Reiki clothing is made from cotton, Lycra, cashmere, silk etc. Other clothes includes tee shirts, denim jackets, tunics, skirts, pants, tank tops and almost all other fashionable forms of clothing. Reiki clothes made from silk are quite popular as it is believed that the properties of silk greatly complement Reiki.

Benefits of Reiki Clothing:

Wearing Reiki clothes has numerous benefits:

1. Balances your body vibrations and revitalizing you from within.

2. Let's you receive enjoy all the benefits of Reiki energy.

3. Helps your body to heal itself.

4. Increases your spirit and energy, and also keeps your energy levels from becoming exhausted.

5. Boosts your confidence and enhances your way of life.

Chapter 14: Reiki Principles: Getting Started With The Five Principles

Over the years, there has been a massive search for the different methods of maximizing human energy with an end goal to control and direct its stream in and around our bodies. Acupuncture (Needle therapy), Feng Shui, Meditation, Tai Chi, and Yoga are among the systems that have been created and used to redirect our energy, with much achievement. And like those antiquated practices, Reiki is a type of hands-on treatment that goes back in history to its starting points in India and the East.

It is another technique that enables the specialist to get to this unadulterated energy and enable it to course through them and treat themselves as well as other people. The first name and procedures were lost because the ancient men conventionally shared information by listening in on others' conversations.

Fortunately, it was re-found by a Japanese priest and researcher named Dr. Mikao Usui who called the procedure "Reiki," signifying "Worldwide Life Force."

Opening energy blockages and empowering this nurturing vitality to flow unrestricted all through the body is the objective of each Reiki treatment.

This all-encompassing methodology works for the body, psyche, and soul to invigorate the body's own normal self-healing capacities.

By permitting the all Universal life power to course through their body, the Reiki specialist goes about as a conductor as they direct this vitality into their customer by means of explicit hand situations.

A person becomes a specialist by regularly performing Reiki within some weeks. This period will help practice and get acquainted with the exercises.

Nonetheless, you can actualize the standards of Reiki into your life promptly and with this, you can change the course of your life.

Reiki is regularly characterized as "Universal Energy" and is a strategy for unwinding dependent on the possibility that cognizant recuperating vitality can be moved through the hands of the professional to the patient.

While Reiki has been accepted as a type of treatment utilized exclusively for healing, it very well may be used to better your regular daily existence, as well.

While there is no incorrect method to actualize these standards into your life, they will serve you best in your adventure of personal development if you endeavor to maintain what they involve.

Try not to be dispirited in the event that you find this hard to do from the start. With enough work on, following these 5 Principles of Reiki will end up easy and you will, before long, have the option to extraordinarily develop yourself.

Anxiety – "Just For Today, I Will Not Worry"

Stress is the main cause of negative energy, which makes this guideline one of the most significant in the 5 Principles of Reiki.

It can corrupt the spirit and soul, and change us into terrible (and undesirable) individuals. Stress can transform us into impolite, irate, restless people. It has the potency of disrupting the harmony between brain, body, and soul.

Executing this mantra into your life will help you understand that at some points, the pressure we feel isn't justified, despite any potential benefits and that it's so much easier to approach every day with an inspirational frame of mind; to set out to remain quiet.

Stress causes pressure and nervousness which prompts an irregularity of the psyche, body and soul.

Mitigate your worry by attempting to see every obstruction in your life as a chance and approach all circumstances with an inspirational frame of mind.

Following this standard is key in personal growth—after some time, you will see a critical lift in your disposition and life will turn out to be quite a lot more charming.

Anger – "Just For Today, I Will Not Be Angry"

Should you consolidate the previous Reiki principle into your life, the subsequences will effortlessly become easy to follow.

Outrage is typically one of the essential side effects of pressure and tension. Obviously, now and then it's an independent negative feeling that burdens us, however in figuring out how to control our stresses, concerns, and responses to others in dealing with our pressure, we figure out how to control different feelings as well.

It is imperative to recall, however, that all forms of negativity, similar to outrage or envy are common: you are not an awful individual for feeling them. It's just that they become hazardous in that they change our conduct, obstruct our affection and light, and corrupt our spirits. In personal development, it is imperative to deal with them, so these feelings don't control us.

Only for now I will not be annoyed: To rehearse this rule, you have to comprehend what triggers your displeasure and how you can control your feelings once more.

At the point when you become furious, the individual or circumstance at that point has unlimited power over you.

When you figure out how to react in a positive way, you will never again enable anything to take your influence and control.

Approach every individual or circumstance with sympathy and attempt to comprehend what is happening underneath the surface.

Try not to harp on negative considerations, and stay around those who have optimistic energy

Diligence – "Just For Today, I Will Do My Work Honestly"

If you think that this principle is all about corruption, then you are wrong. It is not about misleading your manager by telling him that your absence from work is due to illness when you are not, or to abstain from taking the company's stationery.

Even though corruption is also a part, this mantra can be used for more than an ordinary act of honesty.

Handle your work with the expectation of playing out your part as much as you can, and with the objective of imparting the majority of your useful abilities to those you work with.

Do not cheat people by holding any of your natural ability back.

You would likewise be cheating yourself by denying that you have your extraordinary gifts.

Gratitude – "Just For Today, I Will Give Thanks for My Many Blessings"

We come back to the significance of appreciation, regardless of how little our gifts are.

Appreciation could possibly be the most significant blessing people can give. To back it up with scientific facts, appreciation makes us healthy as they make us more joyful and kinder. It is a crucial practice in self-awareness and takes no time or exertion to achieve.

On the off chance that you can't think about any reason to be appreciative, think about the little things. You're alive, you're solid. You have a rooftop over your head, a full stomach, and shoes on your feet.

You can say thank you for a decent climate, or thank you for a decent night's rest. Understanding that every little thing is a blessing will improve your state of mind exponentially. Start by writing an appreciation diary: this is an ideal and powerful approach to actualize this principle into your life!

Take a breath all the time, recognize and welcome the numerous of favors throughout your life.

If you set aside the effort to keep a rundown of your numerous favors, you will, without a doubt, be astonished at what number of brilliant things there are to offer gratitude for.

Don't simply include the temporary materialistic things. Concentrate on the things that cash can't purchase.

Affection – "Just For Today, I Will Be Kind to My Neighbor and Every Living Thing"

Once more, if you practice Principle #4 and figure out how to say thank you, being benevolent will pursue with no exertion by any means.

This (just as appreciation) is ideal for rehearsing mindfulness. At the point when we accomplish beneficial things for other people, it feels great to perceive how we have the ability to make them grin or giggle. Next time you are benevolent to somebody, focus on how they change. It's very enabling and will persuade you to keep doing great.

This equivalent idea applies to animals that are littler than us. All life ought to be regarded. You should, once in a while, try to be benevolent to creatures and perceive how it feels. You could bolster the winged animals at the recreation center, or give nourishment to your nearby creature cover. You don't need to apply so much strength, but it will have any kind of effect to the creatures we regularly overlook.

When rehearsing appreciation and generosity, don't be false about it. It may compensate in the event that you really would not joke about this. Instead of being kind since you trust it will profit you, be benevolent for no other explanation than thoughtfulness itself. Try not to spoil your morals with narrow-mindedness.

What we give, we get, as indicated by Karmic law.

At the point when we think positive contemplations, we carry more things to feel positive about into our lives.

Keep in mind that a similar impact happens when we think of negative contemplations.

Reflecting upon these standards and endeavoring to live inside their structure is sure to impact positive change in all aspects of your life.

For included advantage, plan a Reiki session and experience the full impact of this antiquated all- inclusive principles.

Chapter 15: Basic Reiki Healing Techniques

Reiki healing practices are actually divided into three different lesson levels, each next level consisting of slightly more difficult concepts and techniques than the previous. For the purpose of this guide, we're going to focus on the most basic techniques to help you establish your practice and develop a deeper understanding of the foundations of reiki healing.

37th Thing you need to know...

Your Environment is Key

The efficacy of your reiki healing session will rely on how well you're able to focus your mind on the energy of reiki. If there are any distractions around you - such as physical discomfort, noise, or movement - then you might find it hard to maintain concentration on the task at hand.

For that reason, it's imperative that you optimize your environment to support your reiki healing practice. Here are some elements you might want to consider:

Turn down the lights to a dim glow, as though you were preparing to sleep. Allowing just enough visibility so you can make your way around your space limits the distractions and visual stimulation you perceive during healing.

Find a comfortable spot in your home. Be it a chair or your bed, make sure you're free from discomfort and pain, and that you can maintain your position in your chosen spot for the entire length of healing.

Enhance the mood by lighting a few scented candles or by playing soothing music. The more relaxed and stress-free you feel, the more positive your energy becomes.

Attend to all of your bodily needs. Drink water, relieve yourself, eat, and make sure you're well-rested before you start. Any bodily functions that get in the way of your healing can distract you from your goal and push you to cut your session short.

38th Thing you need to know...

Sense Your Body

The most basic aspect of the reiki healing technique is the process of sensing your body. The full body scan enables you to pick out different sensations throughout your body. The purpose of the scan is to determine where you should focus your healing energy.

This part of the process ties in with intention setting. If you want to use reiki healing for the purpose of physical wellness, then you may want to consider scanning your body before you set your intention. Doing so will help you target the areas that need the most attention.

Another benefit of the full body scan is that it enables you to reveal the truth of your life force. Not everyone is deeply attuned to their energy, and so it might be a challenge to fully understand when you're making an actual impact on your life force by way of reiki. Taking the time to 'sense' the energy in your body will help you attune to its properties and become more sensitive to changes, improvements, and blockages that it might manifest.

To start the full body scan, follow these steps:

Lie down and try to achieve a state of mindfulness.

Once in a mindful, meditative state, close your eyes and sense the toes on your feet. How do they feel? Can you visualize the energy flowing through them? Do you sense any blockages? Ask yourself these questions for each new part you progress to.

Work your way slowly and deliberately from your feet, up to your knees, your thighs, until you reach the crown of your head. Always ask yourself the previous questions in order to properly investigate the status of the energy in that body part.

Any areas where there might be a blockage should be remembered. Make a mental note of the parts of your body where you sense a potential disturbance.

Throughout the process, do not attempt to change anything. If it happens that there's a blockage in a part of your body, don't attempt to release the tension just yet.

The objective of the full body scan is not to heal but to help you understand where you should direct your healing energy.

39th Thing you need to know...

The Basic Reiki Hand Positions

There are an infinite number of hand positions in the reiki healing practice, each of which aims to target the different problems and ailments that people might experience. For this basic instruction, we're focusing on 15 different basic reiki hand positions that may come in handy as you learn the ropes.

These hand positions have no inherent meaning other than the fact that they aim to imbibe positive healing energy where it might be necessary. As the healer, it is up to you whether you feel more empowered when you touch the parts being addressed, or if you simply hover your hands over the target area. There is no right or wrong way.

Position 1 - Over the face with the fingers touching over the forehead

Position 2 - Over the head with fingers touching along the midline of the skull

Position 3 - Cupping the ears, with the fingers resting on the temples of the forehead

Position 4 - Along the nape, with the tips of the fingers touching gently

Position 5 - Over the shoulders, with the pinky side of the hand touching the neck

Position 6 - Just under the ribs, with the tips of the fingers touching

Position 7 - At the level of the belly button, fingers touching

Position 8 - At the level of the pubic bone, fingers touching

Position 9 - On the lower back just above the buttocks, fingers touching

Position 10 - Slightly higher on the lower back, over the sacral area, fingers touching

Position 11 - Bend down and hold the left foot with both hands

Position 12 - Bend down and hold the right foot with both hands

Position 13 - Bend down and hold the right foot with the right hand, and the left foot with the left hand simultaneously

40th Thing you need to know...

More Than Just Touching

These basic hand techniques don't only encourage you to touch your different body parts. There is a deep cognitive facet to these techniques, requiring the full participation of your mind and spirit in order to be truly effective in offering you healing.

During each step of the process, repeat your mantra and remind yourself why you're undergoing healing in the first place. Remember the areas of your body that piqued your interest during the full body scan that you performed prior to healing.

Every step of the way, try to maximize the feeling capabilities of your hands. Focus on the healing energy passing through them. Feel the warmth of your hands and visualize the energy in your system as you move along. In the areas of blockage, imaging the energy repairing damage and encouraging the ideal vibration and vigor where it might have been lost. Repeat to yourself, "I am a child of the universe, and I deserve to heal."

41st Thing you need to know...

The Possibilities are Endless

Even with these basic hand techniques, the possibilities of healing are endless. Using a combination of these hand gestures, or using them in sequence, can help you target a variety of problems. Remember, the key to an effective reiki healing practice doesn't rely on how well you follow rules and sequences, but on how well you're able to satisfy what feels right for your body.

42nd Thing you need to know...

There is No Single Right Way to Do It

Create your own healing sequences and follow what your body tells you. Be attuned with your system and truly feel what your body needs. The better you know your own body and the deeper you connect with your life force, the easier it becomes to use reiki healing.

Chapter 16: Chakras In The Context

Of Reiki

The hand placements used in Reiki healing usually target the seven major chakras as well as the secondary chakras, which are also important. The secondary chakras are often dysfunctional and discolored, and sometimes even completely closed, due to problems in the mind, body or spirit. Being able to keep the chakras functioning properly is very important to one's health because disruptions in energy flow cause illness. In this chapter, we will discuss the concept of the chakra in Reiki, as well as the different chakras and what they have an effect on.

What is the Chakra?

The term Chakra originated in the ancient Indian language of Sanskrit. It literally means vortex, spinning wheel, or circle. The chakras turn in a clockwise direction and resemble a spinning fan. Each individual chakra spins at its own frequency, which allows the ki, or the universal life force, to be drawn into the body, keeping the physical, mental, emotional and spiritual elements of the body healthy and balanced. When releasing unwanted ki or dealing with other people or situations, the chakras spin outwards.

Chakras are the channels through which energy enters and leaves our bodies, both physically and of the aura. They are found within every level of our aura, physical, mental, emotional and spiritual, so they affect every part of the being. This means that when we have good feelings, such as relaxation and happiness, our chakras are spinning openly and evenly, which creates a balanced aura that is well protected. However, when we are feeling depresion, anxiety, stress, and other similar emotions, then the chakras will be depleted and this will also affect our aura. Over time, these negative emotions can drain the chakra completely and begin to affect one's well being, and this is where Reiki healing comes in.

The worry and stress that come naturally as a part of our daily lives causes blockages in our energy centers. Holding on to negative thoughts causes our chakras to become tainted with dense energy and this in turn has a constricting effect on the flow of energy through our chakras, which is the root of the sluggish, or unbalanced feeling that people often get. A block is a place where energy has become trapped due to this, and Reki gets the energy moving in order to deal with a block. As the energy flows through the whole body, it replaces dissonance and imbalance with harmony, and helping to bring the chakras into alignment and balance them.

Each chakra is a part of the entire energy system, so no one chakra works independently of the others. An individual chakra can only work fully when the others are also fully engaged. Each of them as a role that balances an aspect of our life, whether it is physical, emotional, mental or spiritual. Thus it is essential in maintaining good health to know whether or not our chakras are balanced and if not, how unbalanced they are.

The Seven Chakras

There are seven main chakras. The first three deal with physical and material issues, and are often termed the lower chakras. the other four, from the heart chakra up, have to do with spiritual issues, and are called upper chakras.

Root Chakra: The Spirit of Life

The root chakra can be found at the base of the spine, and it is an element of our foundation. It represents earth and has a direct correlation to our survival instincts, or the need for food, shelter and protection. It also activates the urge for us to take care of ourselves and defend ourselves in order to maintain life. In addition, it appeals to the sens of grounding and connection that we have with our physical bodies and physical world. When fully functioning, this chakra brings a sense of security and presence.

This chakra is associated with the color red, and is linked to the adrenal glands, kidneys, spinal column and leg bones.

When this chakra becomes imbalanced, one can become afraid of life, withdrawing from physical reality and sustaining feelings of victimization. It can also cause selfish actions and vulnerability to violence. Imbalance of this chakra can also cause problems in the feet, legs, and lower back.

Sacral Chakra: The Spirit of Health and Purity

This chakra, the sacral chakra, is located in the abdomen, lower back and sexual organs. It is associated with the color orange. It is related to the element of water, and controls our emotions and sexuality. It works to provide a sense of one's inner self or inner child. It is also the place from which creativity and inspiration stems. It controls our cravings for sensation, whether they be sound, smell, taste, touch or sight. When working properly, this chakra brings depth of feeling, as well as sexual fulfillment and the ability to accept change.

The parts of the body which the sacral chakra are related to are the gonads, the prostate gland, the reproductive system, the spleen and the bladder. An imbalance in this chakra can cause over indulgence in sex or food, as well as sexual or reproductive disorders and feelings of jealousy and confusion. Self esteem issues can also be negatively or positively affected by this center of energy.

The Solar Plexus Chakra: The Spirit of Knowledge and Wisdom

Associated with the color yellow, the solar plexus chakra is also called the power chakra, and is located at the solar plexus. It mainly functions as a means of supply energy in the form of heat, power and enthusiasm. It rules the consciousness of decision, creative expression, personal power, will and autonomy. It can even have an effect on one's metabolism. When this chakra is balanced, it brings energy, effectiveness and spontaneity. It also allows one to become aware of the divine guidance flowing into one's life.

This chakra is connected to the pancreas, liver, digestive tract, stomach, spleen, gall bladder and autonomic nervous system. It is also strongly connected to intellect, and is the seat of our personal power. The energy of this chakra can help to turn one's hopes and dreams into reality, and allow self confidence and a clear sense of direction and purpose in one's life. Problems in this chakra can cause insecurity about physical and financial matters and the necessity to dominate other people. Physical problems which can stem from the imbalance of this chakra can include digestive disorders.

The Heart Chakra: The Spirit of Evolution

The heart chakra is connected to the color green, and is located directly at the center of the chest. It is directly related to love and compassion and links the lower or physical self to the higher or spiritual self.

The balanced state of our fourth chakra allows for one to love deeply, feel compassion and feel peace and centeredness. It is the center of love and emotional well being and develops our ablity to both give and receive unconditional love when it is functioning at its best.

When it is not however, one can experience feelings of sadness, fear and anger. The heart chakra is related to the thymus gland, the heart, the lower lungs, the circulatory system and the skin and hands. When it is not working properly, it can result in heart disease.

The Throat Chakra: The Spirit of Truth and Expression

The throat chakra is identified with the color blue, and is related to communication, as well as creativity and self expression. It allows for free communication which helps us to feel centered and happy. It also helps to guide meditation, allowing for connection with our higher guidance. It is connected deeply to the soul and inner self and allows us to listen as our soul speaks. When the throat chakra is working optimally, it can allow us to speak and listen in the spirit of truth as well as constructively express our anger and other emotions, both negative and positive. Adding energy to this chakra can help to improve psychic ability.

The throat chakra is linked to the thyroid gland, throat and jaw area, vocal chords and digestive tract. When it is blocked, communication suffers, and one may overindulge in eating and drinking in an attempt to distract from a non communicative throat. This can cause respiratory diseases, dental disorders and low self esteem. Feelings of anger, hostility and resentment are also linked to the poor functioning of this chakra.

The Third Eye Chakra: The Spirit of Clarity and Psychic Awareness

The third eye chakra, which is indigo, is also known as the brow chakra. It is located slightly above and between the eye brows. It mainly works as the center of inner vision and is the place of intuition and soul knowledge. It allows for the opening of psychic and spiritual awareness and causes understanding of archetypal levels. A balanced third eye chakra allows for insight and knowledge.

This chakra is associated with the pituitary gland, lower brain, left eye, ears, nose and central nervous system. This is the chakra which is susceptible to the most blockage. Blockage of the third eye chakra leads to fear of the imagination, dreams and irrational thought. In the physical body, an imbalance of one's third eye can cause persistent headaches, as well as insomnia, anxiety and depression.

The Crown Chakra

The crown chakra is linked to the color violet and relates to consciousness as pure awareness. It is located at the top of the head and represents our connection to the collective consciousness and the world beyond. It is widely believed that this is where the soul enters the body at birth and departs at the time of one's death. When it is balanced and well developed, it can bring knowledge, wisdom, understanding, spiritual connection and harmony. A highly developed crown chakra also allows one to understand the "oneness" of universal existence and experience true inner peace, removing the separation between ourselves and other beings.

Expanding the crown chakra allows us to have access to the highest sources of spiritual wisdom as well as enhance our psychic knowing. This chakra is related physically to the pineal gland, upper brain and right eye. When it is blocked it results in feelings of loneliness, fear of death and a need to compare ourselves to others.

Chapter 17: Breathing: It Really Is Important!

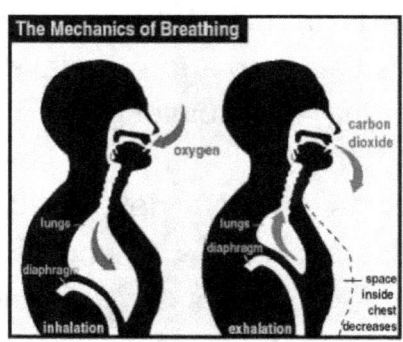

Just sit where you are. If you're in a straight backed chair, lift your chin so it's parallel to the floor and pull your shoulders back just a little to align your spine and open your rib cage and abdomen. Let your hands rest on your thighs as you maintain that position and just relax your muscles as much as you can. Now close your eyes.

Inhale through your nose for a count of four: one-one thousand, two-one thousand, three-one thousand, four-one thousand. Some people can inhale longer than four seconds. If you are one of those lucky people, inhale as you count the seconds until you can't inhale any more.

Feel how your shoulders lift as you pull that breath in. Feel your rib cage expanding, the cartilage between those slender bones stretching as you fill your lungs. Feel the way your abdominal muscles relax to allow full expansion of your lungs. Feel your diaphragm drop and loosen.

Now slowly exhale through your mouth until you feel like your lungs are empty, usually a count of eight. And repeat.

Feel how your diaphragm contracts to expel the air in your lungs. Feel your abdominal muscles tighten to maintain your upright posture. Feel the way your rib cage collapses gently around your deflating lungs, the slender bones cradling those infinitely important organs protectively. Feel your shoulders roll slightly on each exhale as tension eases in your neck, shoulders, upper arms and upper back.

Now, open your eyes. Did you feel it? Wasn't it amazing? It is extraordinary to know that your body does that every day of your life from the day you are born to the day you die without having to consciously think about it. But when you do think about it and take the time to feel it – it's absolutely mind-blowing!

Most people feel light-headed after a few minutes of this deep breathing; this is normal. Your body doesn't breathe as deeply when you are tense or active. Only when you are relaxed can you breathe as deeply as your body needs. You may feel a slight tingling in your extremities and this too is normal as more oxygen than your fingers and toes are used to is being sent to those capillaries.

Would you be surprised to find out you just centered yourself? Yes, it is true. You just centered yourself with that simple deep breathing method. In the same way that those who meditate begin their meditations.

This is the first step to learning Reiki for yourself. This sort of deep breathing and concentrating on how that air flows into your lungs and the mild relaxation and clarity of mind it offers. The next step is often the most fun, but can also be the most difficult for some people.

Chapter 18: The Chakras, Meridians

And Also Reiki

Chakras are facilities of spiritual power situated at certain factors in the physical body based on Yoga exercise viewpoint. Chakras are made up of refined physical body levels that follower out in the form of a heart. The 7 primary Chakras (there are small ones additionally) give off a light as well as are thought to stay in our refined or spiritual physical body.

2. Sacral chakra (linked shade: orange; relevant components of the physical body: gonads, prostrate glandular, reproductive system, spleen, bladder).

When effectively working, this chakra energies our feelings, imagination as well as sexuality. We really feel important and also casual, all set to confiscate the minute. Discrepancy of this chakra could cause over-indulgence in sex or food, sex-related or reproductive problems, as well as sensations of envy and also complication.

3. Solar plexus chakra (connected shade: yellow; associated components of the physical body: pancreatic, liver, digestive system system, tummy, spleen, gall bladder, free nerve system).

Highly connected with intelligence, the solar plexus chakra is likewise the seat of our individual power. Disorder of this chakra could result in instability concerning physical as well as monetary concerns as well as the requirement to control others.

4. Heart chakra (linked shade: environment-friendly (additional shade: pink); relevant components of the physical body: thymus glandular, heart, reduced lungs, blood circulation system, skin, hands).

When this chakra is operating efficiently, our capacity to offer as well as get genuine love is well created. Disorder of this chakra typically results in sensations of despair, anxiety as well as temper and also could lead to heart condition.

5. Throat chakra (connected shade: sky blue; associated components of the physical body: thyroid glandular, throat and also mouth locations, lungs, singing cables, digestion system).

Stimulating this chakra could enhance our psychic hearing capability called clairaudience. Normally, interaction experiences when this chakra is obstructed. Sensations of temper, hostility as well as bitterness additionally are linked with the discrepancy of this chakra.

6. Third-eye chakra (connected shade: indigo; associated components of the physical body: pituitary glandular, reduced human brain, left eye, ears, nose, main nerve system).

An open third-eye chakra is the resource of our instinct and also clairvoyance (vision past normal view) in addition to our capability to picture as well as materialize. Clogs of this chakra are plentiful, leading to worry of the creative imagination, fantasizes and also our "illogical" instinctive understandings. Physical signs of third-eye inequality might consist of relentless migraines (specifically in the facility of the temple), sleeping disorders, stress and anxiety as well as anxiety.

7. Crown chakra (connected shade: violet (likewise white); associated components of the physical body: pineal glandular, top human brain, best eye).

The crown chakra is our straight link to spirit. Development of the crown chakra allows us to touch right into the greatest resources of spiritual knowledge and also boost our claircognizance (psychic recognizing).

I provided the Crown Chakra as 7 a great deal of attunements really begin with that Chakra initially as well as go down from there. With the Base Chakra last. According to conventional writing, over 88,000 Chakras cover basically every component of our physical bodies.

It streams right into your physical body via your crown as well as heart chakras as well as out with your hand chakras to anywhere you route it (to certain components of your physical body or to others).

The origin and also crown chakras could be thought about paired due to the fact that they are the flexible factors of the physical body's primary power existing, which runs up as well as down the spinal column and also right into which all of the chakras factor

The chakras transform power from one degree to one more by dispersing Ki (likewise called Chi, Prana, Mana depending on idea system) to the physical body. Well balanced origin chakras result in a healthy and balanced need for the fundamentals of life (food, heat, sanctuary, and so on) When this chakra is unbalanced, we could be worried of life, take out from physical fact, really feel taken advantage of, run in an extremely self-centered method, or be susceptible to physical violence. I noted the Crown Chakra as 7 a great deal of attunements in fact begin with that Chakra initially as well as go down from there.

They are the facilities that share and also obtain the vital force power. They send and also obtain powers to and also from deep space, nature, holy beings and also various other living points as well as sometimes-inanimate items.

Prior to an individual has a Reiki attunement, an ordinary individual's mood might just prolong an only a few decimeters from an individual's physical body. Via the Reiki attunement and also the fortifying of the mood you obtain the power tool to take control over your life and also growth.

Throughout a Reiki therapy, not just the body organs as well as the power circulation within the physical body are influenced however likewise the various physical bodies of the mood are impacted. When utilizing range recovery or the mental/emotional sign the mood appears to be much more damaged compared to the real body organs in the physical body.

BLUE MOOD SHADE: Connects to the throat, thyroid. Great, tranquil, as well as gathered. Caring, caring, love to aid others, delicate, user-friendly.

Soft blue: Serenity, clearness as well as interaction; genuine; instinctive.

Intense royal blue: Clairvoyant; extremely spiritual nature; charitable; on the best course; brand-new chances are coming.

Dark or sloppy blue: Anxiety of the future; worry of self-expression; anxiety of encountering or consulting the reality.

YELLOW MOOD SHADE: Connects to the spleen and also life power. It is the shade of awakening, motivation, knowledge as well as activity discussed, imaginative, lively, positive, as well as carefree.

Light or light yellow: Arising psychic as well as spiritual understanding; positive outlook and also hopefulness; favorable enjoyment concerning originalities.

Brilliant lemon-yellow: Battling to preserve power as well as control in an individual or company partnership; anxiety of blowing up, stature, regard, and/or power.

Clear gold metal, glossy as well as intense: Spiritual power as well as power triggered as well as stired up; an influenced individual.

Dark brown yellow or gold: A pupil, or one that is stressing at examining; extremely logical to the factor of sensation worn down or worried; aiming to offset "lost time" by discovering every little thing simultaneously.

Do completely dry showering (Kenyoku) to separate from their power area. Kenyoku implies "completely dry showering" as well as is a strategy for routine filtration utilizing power instead compared to water. It could likewise be made use of at different times via the day or anytime one really feels the requirement to launch adverse power.

Standard Gassho is straightforward, rest with your hands in petition placement (Gassho implies petition placement) as well as focus on breathing in and also out gradually. With each in breath picture that Reiki is entering your crown as well as loading your whole physical body - with each outbreath picture that you are breathing out Reiki from every pore in your physical body and also off out right into infinity. Exercise Gassho day-to-day for 10-15 mins till you are made use of to it.

2. Put your right-hand man on your left shoulder.

3. Brush down your breast, throughout your tummy as well as end at the appropriate hip.

4. Do the very same beyond.

5. Repeat action # 2.

6. Expand your left arm.

7. Rub down your arm completely to the hand as well as finger pointers. Fling your best hand out right into the air as though you are tossing away any sort of adverse power.

8. Do the exact same with the ideal arm.

9. Repeat the stroke down the left arm once more.

10. You could do a brief Gassho once more if you want.

ECO-FRIENDLY MOOD SHADE: Associates to heart and also lungs. When seen in the mood this normally stands for development and also equilibrium, and also many of all, something that leads to alter.

Intense emerald environment-friendly: A therapist, additionally a love-centered individual.

Yellow-Green: Imaginative with heart, communicative.

Dark or sloppy woodland environment-friendly: Envy, animosity, seeming like a sufferer of the globe; criticizing self or others; instability as well as reduced self-worth; absence of comprehending individual duty; conscious regarded objection.

Blue-green: Associates with the body immune system. Delicate, thoughtful, therapist, specialist.

INDIGO MOOD SHADE: Associates with the 3rd eye, aesthetic as well as pituitary glandular. Instinctive, delicate, deep sensation.

VIOLET MOOD SHADE: Associates to crown, pineal glandular and also stressed system. This is the instinctive shade in the mood, as well as discloses psychic power of attunement with self.

LAVENDER MOOD SHADE: Creative imagination, visionary, daydreamer, etheric.

SILVER MOOD SHADE: This is the shade of wealth, both spiritual and also physical. Bunches of intense silver could mirror to lots of cash, and/or awakening of the planetary mind.

Intense metal silver: Responsive to originalities; instinctive; supporting.

Dark as well as sloppy grey: Deposit of anxiety is gathering in the physical body, with a possibility for health issue, specifically if grey collections seen in particular locations of the physical body.

GOLD MOOD SHADE: The shade of knowledge as well as magnificent defense. When seen within the mood, it states that the individual is being directed by their greatest excellent.

BLACK MOOD SHADE: Attracts or draws power to it and also in so doing, changes it. It catches light and also eats it. Generally shows lasting unforgiveness (towards others or an additional) gathered in a particular location of the physical body, which could cause health issue; additionally, bodies within an individual's mood, chakras, or physical body; previous life injures; unreleased sorrow from abortions if it shows up in the ovaries.

WHITE MOOD SHADE: Shows various other power. Frequently stands for a brand-new, not yet assigned power in the mood.

White glimmers or flashes of white light: angels neighbor; could show that the individual is expectant or will certainly be quickly.

PLANET MOOD SHADES: Dirt, timber, mineral, plant. These shades present a love of the Planet, of being based and also is seen in those that live and also work with the outdoors ... building, farming, and so on. These shades are very important as well as are a great indication.

RAINBOWS: Rainbow-colored red stripes, standing out like sunbeams from the hand, head or physical body: A Reiki therapist, or a celebrity individual (an individual that remains in the very first manifestation in the world).

PASTELS: A delicate mix of light as well as shade, compared to standard shades. Reveals level of sensitivity and also a requirement for calmness.

FILTHY BROWN OVERLAY: Holding on powers. Instability.

UNCLEAN GRAY EXTREMELY: Obstructing powers. Guardedness.

In our everyday lives our moods go through numerous undesirable resonances. Harmful resonance consist of such points as electro-magnetic resonance from digital gadgets, toxins, or even our adverse feelings. Also an individual routing unfavorable power at you could contaminate your mood.

This method will certainly brush your physical body mood as well as make it prepared to get Reiki resonance. When one does not wash the mood initially it makes it harder for the Reiki job to permeate.

Clearing up the Mood is a pre-healing device in as well as of itself. To cleanse somebody's mood the recipient could either exist or rest easily.

The specialist does brushing motions regarding 10 centimeters far from the one obtaining the cleaning. This could be done from head to toe or from left to. The mood will certainly obtain readjusted in this manner and also the excess power streams off of the hands of the expert as they send out readjusting power to the individuals mood.

After a Reiki therapy blog post mood cleaning is really crucial. The last mood cleaning shuts the chakras and also mood so it will certainly not get any kind of undesirable power once the individual is well balanced. The specialist would certainly execute the blog post mood cleansing in the very same means they did the pre cleansing.

The mood is composed of 7 levels or degrees called auric physical bodies. This parallels with the 7 major Chakras which stem in the human physical body however additionally already exist in the degrees of the mood. A state of discrepancy in one of the physical bodies leads to a state of discrepancy in the various other.

The 7 auric levels or physical bodies are:

The Physical body- This is where the physical feelings obtain from. The physical body is the most concrete symptom of our awareness. We all understand the anxieties of the physical body - illness, aging and also fatality.

The Etheric physical body- This is where the power is shown when it moves via meridians and also chakras. The etheric physical body or dual acts as a design template for the physical body as well as shows up as a power matrix. It is explained in Chinese medication as meridians that send Qi/Ki with the physical body.

Range recovery component of mood cleaning while doing Reiki. (You could do the actions on yourself listed below as well to offer on your own a therapy when required or prior to you send out Reiki to a person else).

Picture the individual you are to function on. You desire to attempt and also send out the range recovery for regarding 10 to 20 mins for every degree of being.

The light power goes inside from that factor and also loads their whole physical body up gradually. As their physical body loads with the Power their whole entire internal physical body is being filled up and also bordered consisting of the body organs with power. The power needs to emit to the exterior of the receivers physical body.

Visualize that the radiance from their physical body currently expands out right into their psychological degree. Utilizing the proper Chakra like the heart, solarplex and also navel and also the etheric auric physical body as well as the Celestial physical body.

Think of that fear delicately streams out of their physical body. As all these unpleasant ideas leave their physical body, Reiki loads up as well as expands out right into their psychological degree. You could send this to the Essential, Reduced as well as Greater Auric physical bodies as well as the matching Chakras.

Picture it as a gorgeous gold circulation of power that is a straight web link to the greater worlds. Mean that the Reiki power reconnects them to the divine within them as well as reignites their fire. See them loaded with spiritual power that prolongs out past all the various other degrees of their being.

The etheric physical body or dual acts as a design template for the physical body as well as shows up as a power matrix. Psychological Physical body or Celestial Psychological Physical body- This auric physical body offers to educate us self-knowledge. The Causal physical body (Ketheric Design template) or the Spiritual Instinctive Physical body- The powers in this physical body rotates with an extremely high regularity. Generally suggests lasting unforgiveness (towards others or an additional) accumulated in a particular location of the physical body, which could lead to wellness troubles; likewise, bodies within an individual's mood, chakras, or physical body; previous life harms; unreleased despair from abortions if it shows up in the ovaries.

As their physical body loads with the Power their whole entire internal physical body is being loaded as well as bordered liking the body organs with power.

Chapter 19: Other Self-Healing

Techniques

What Is Healing Touch?

Unlike Reiki, before you can exercise it, Healing Touch does not involve a tuning. It is a modality that Janet Mentgen, R.N. has created. And it was for those in the medical sector initially. It's accessible to all, though. It's a modality of energy, like Reiki. Several concentrations exist. Level I based on 15 or more clock hours of training that enables individuals of different backgrounds to join, recognize their prior learning and further develop energy-based treatment ideas and abilities. There is also a need for powerful personal growth engagement and an understanding of holistic health values. Between these concentrations, there is no necessary waiting period, and they can teach each weekend, it is vital to have a knowledge of the 12 meridians and the chakras in healing touch, also known as therapeutic touch, and to learn

hands-on therapeutic abilities in opening blocked energies. It needs mild practitioner-to-receiver use of hands. For particular circumstances such as back issues, Healing Touch has more methods available. Healing Touch is a way to change the energy system of the body in order to impact self-healing.

What Is Reiki?

Reiki channels the universal life energy is known as qi to boost mental, body, and spirit integration to improve the natural healing system. A Buddist Monk named Mikao Usui developed it in 1922. He taught the exercise to over 2,000 students before his death. Reiki can generally be trained in a weekend like Healing Touch. While many organizations give practitioners certificates, these courses are not formally regulated.

Before they can exercise on others, Reiki practitioners must be aligned. If the qi of the practitioner is blocked, their healing abilities will be hindered. The strokes in Reiki are comparable to those observed in Healing Touch but are performed near the body, not directly on the body. This could create Reiki for those who dislike being touched a more comfortable exercise.

The Difference Between Healing Touch and Reiki

Healing Touch and Reiki are comparable alternative medicines, but the two differ significantly. Both are regarded as a form of alternative medicine known as energy medicine. Blocked energies can be published in both Healing Touch and Reiki that can assist promote the healing of many fundamental illnesses and illnesses. The concept behind both is that the physician can channel the patient's life energy to encourage the process of healing to start. Many think these procedures encourage the body to heal itself without any additional medical intervention.

Although there are no clinical findings to demonstrate these allegations, the results of Reiki and Healing Touch swear by many patients.

Incorporating Reiki Healing into Your Yoga Practice

Guess what's missing from your yoga practice? (Hint: Reiki)

You've got a dozen yoga mats, a few stylish yoga outfits, and a few props. Your previous courses of yoga, books, and videos make sure you have down patted your poses and sequences. But as you advanced along your yoga trip, you may have begun to feel that something was missing from your exercise at home, something that could bring you to a greater, more enlightened plane.

That something you're lacking maybe that thing called Reiki.

Reiki Healing and Life Force Energy

Reiki is an ancient Japanese healing method that includes transferring "life force energy" or prana to particular areas of the body by laying hands on it. Reiki masters have effectively unlocked their prana free flow and can transfer Reiki's capacity to learners through a method known as "attunement." Once your own prana is unlocked and you have the capacity to use Reiki, you can use it on others or yourself, concentrating the energy of life force on particular areas of the body that can assist cure wounds and encourage excellent general health and wellbeing.

There are several including Yoga, Tai chi, Ayurveda, Acupuncture, Reflexology, Qi Do, Qi Gong, therapeutic touch, Bioresonance, and acupressure. Depending on what you are looking for may determine which of these (or others) you choose to techniques! Reiki is common because learning and mastering are simple. Qi Gong, Qi Do, and other comparable arts are more difficult because you need to construct your private energy to work with others.

Yoga For Unity and Balance

The practice is much more than just a workout, despite the popular misconception that yoga is a type of exercise. This ancient discipline originated in India, and the term ' yoga' means' joughing' or'uniting.' Yoga enables one to unite body and mind at a fundamental stage. Yoga tries to unite the person with the universal at a deeper level. Yoga teaches you how to relax and release tension, and how to reinforce and stretch stiff muscles. It also helps balance and integrates mind, body, and spirit increases power flow and boosts the natural healing procedures of the body itself. Yoga approaches wellness in a holistic way as a strong form of mind-body medicine, acknowledging that physical ailments also have mental and spiritual elements. Yoga is an extensive self-development and transformation scheme at its core.

- Stress relief. As scientific studies have found, yoga lowers heart rates, reduces blood pressure, and decreases the production of stress hormones such as cortisol. High levels of cortisol are linked to depression, osteoporosis, and abdominal weight gain.

- Greater immune function. Yoga's postures improve the flow of the lymphatic system, responsible for fighting infection and releasing toxins from the body.

- Flexibility and balance. Yoga helps release tight muscles and increase range of

motion. Even those who claim to be "genetically inflexible" are surprised to find how much more limber they can become through a regular yoga practice. Yoga also deepens your awareness of your body, allowing you to improve your balance and posture.

- Strength. Yoga is a powerful strength-building exercise for every part of the body, including the muscles of your core, back, legs, chest, and arms. This helps prevent problems such as back pain and arthritis. As you strengthen your body, you also build your inner strength, discipline, and self-confidence.

- Improved mood. Yoga balances the central nervous system and endocrine system and stimulates the release of endorphins – natural mood-elevating neurochemicals. As you practice, your mind relaxes and you're able to stop dwelling on stressful thoughts and situations, as said by Chopra in Yoga can Heal Your Life, 2019.

Conclusion

We're finally at the end of the book. From the meaning to the techniques, you have learned what Reiki is and how it can be beneficial for you. It may have a bit of a tricky history and a mixed reception worldwide, especially with the many naysayers out there, but as you have learned, a lot of people think that it has allowed them to feel better and refreshed. Others can even say that the pain they once felt is gone because of it. They even get better sleep, too. And many have also integrated Reiki so well into their lives that they have ascended through the levels, got their attunements, and become practitioners themselves. Thus, they can share what they have learned with others.

Reiki has also been a great healing method. Even when the techniques are a bit challenging to do, they have turned into natural skills as time has passed by and revealed that energy can be cultivated with patience and perseverance. Even the simple act of meditation has become a growing trend in the world of Reiki.

Furthermore, Reiki healing is not just about the techniques themselves. It is also about fulfilling principles, being open to everyone, knowing that within ourselves is the energy we've all had right from the start, integrating the essence of the symbols that represent Reiki, and sharing what we have learned to everyone else who needs it.

After all, who would have thought that a rich doctor who went on a 21-day fast would envision the symbols that would build up the foundation for Reiki? With what Dr. Mikao Usui taught his students, his legacy for cultivating energy has lived on. Since then, it has touched many lives, built different types, branched out to everyone from all religions, and provided a new kind of light to millions of people.

Still, do not think that ascending to the highest Reiki level entails that your journey is over. No, it has only just begun. You will find the path towards learning more about Reiki and how it will benefit and bring you wonders that you have never thought possible in your life. It is also a way to see that Reiki has evolved.

Eventually, you may realize that Reiki is not just a healing method that you can learn and master: It can also be a lifestyle that will help you cultivate the energy you have waited for so long to have. It will be a way for you to carve a new path with opportunities and show you that you can control your fate.

You may not be able to control everything in life, but if you can channel the energy on the things you can, it will fill you up with the kind of light that you will never forget. Reiki can show you that deep within your heart is a light that you can use to heal yourself and others.

So, what are you waiting for? Go for it, practice Reiki techniques, and feel the energy flow from within!

www.ingramcontent.com/pod-product-compliance
Lightning Source LLC
Chambersburg PA
CBHW072003070526
44583CB00015B/1307